T0032478

How to Respond Better to the Next Pandemic

THE TANNER LECTURES
ON HUMAN VALUES

How to Respond Better to the Next Pandemic

Remedying Institutional Failures

Allen Buchanan
with commentaries by
Cécile Fabre
Paul Tucker

Foreword by
Mark Matheson

THE UNIVERSITY OF UTAH PRESS
Salt Lake City

Copyright © 2024 by The University of Utah Press. All rights reserved.

Library of Congress Cataloging-in-Publication Data

Names: Buchanan, Allen E., 1948- author.
Title: How to respond better to the next pandemic : remedying institutional failures / Allen
    Buchanan.
Other titles: Tanner lectures on human values
Identifiers: LCCN 2023037524 | ISBN 9781647691691 (paperback) | ISBN 9781647691707
    (ebook)
Subjects: LCSH: COVID-19 (Disease)—Government policy—United States. | COVID-19
    Pandemic, 2020—Government policy—United States. | Pandemics—Government
    policy—United States. | Pandemics—United States—Prevention. | Emergency
    management—United States. | COVID-19 (Disease)—Government policy. | COVID-19
    Pandemic, 2020—Government policy. | Pandemics—Government policy. | Pandemics—
    Prevention. | Emergency management.
Classification: LCC RA644.C67 B828 2023 | DDC 362.1962/4144—dc23/eng/20231101
LC record available at https://lccn.loc.gov/2023037524

∞ This symbol indicates books printed on paper that meets the minimum requirements of
American National Standard for Information Services—Permanence of Paper for Printed
Library Materials, ANSI A39.38\-1984.

Interior printed on recycled paper with 50% post-consumer content.

CONTENTS

FOREWORD

Obert and Grace Tanner envisioned the Tanner Lectures during a walk in their beloved Southern Utah in 1975. The program, as it approaches its fiftieth anniversary, has become the leading academic lecture series in the world. Annual Tanner Lectures are given at nine universities: Stanford, Berkeley, Utah, Michigan, Harvard, Princeton, Yale, Oxford, and Cambridge. Individual Lectures are also sponsored at other domestic and international centers of learning. Obert Tanner once wrote that the purpose of the Tanner Lectures is to contribute to "the moral and intellectual life" of humankind, and for almost half a century the program has provided a forum for eminent scholars, writers, artists, and political leaders.

Following the disruption caused by the COVID-19 pandemic, the Tanner Lectures program is energetically moving forward. In-person Lectures are once again being given, and they continue to function in accordance with the hope of the founders, as lively moments of community building in which ideas are shared and richer futures imagined.

A fresh approach is also being taken in the publication of the Tanner Lectures. The annual volume, in which the Lectures of a given academic year are collected, will remain a central feature of the program. But the administration of the Lectures is also exploring, with its longtime partner the University of Utah Press, flexible and creative ways of making the Lectures more broadly available, in multiple forms, to a worldwide audience.

From the beginning, a favored plan for Tanner Lecture events has involved convening additional scholars to evaluate the Lecture and to participate in discussion and debate with the speaker. In the current volume, the Tanner Lectures is publishing a study by Allen Buchanan, Professor at Duke University and the University of Arizona, which developed from his Tanner Lectures at Clare Hall at the University of Cambridge in 2022. Also included are commentaries from the two respondents on that occasion, Cécile Fabre, Professor of Political Philosophy at Oxford, and Paul Tucker, Fellow of the Kennedy School and the Center for European Studies at Harvard. The publication thus represents a Tanner event involving a colloquy among scholars, but with this difference: Buchanan, clearly compelled by his timely topic of how we might best prepare for the next pandemic, has expanded his analysis to a book-length volume. Both Fabre and Tucker have had access to Buchanan's completed manuscript, and their comments reflect their knowledge of this larger project.

The current volume also represents the full return to vigorous Tanner publishing following the pause imposed by the pandemic. As we move forward with the publication of the Lectures, I'm particularly grateful for the guidance and expertise of Glenda Cotter, the director and editor in chief of the University of Utah Press. I also want to thank Alan Short, President of Clare Hall and Professor Emeritus at Cambridge, for his numerous contributions to this volume and to the Tanner Lectures. Making the content of the Lectures widely available was a fundamental part of Obert's original vision, and the program remains wholly dedicated to this goal as it approaches its fiftieth anniversary.

MARK MATHESON
Director, The Tanner Lectures on
Human Values

ACKNOWLEDGMENTS

I am deeply indebted to the Tanner Foundation for the honor of being selected to deliver the 2022 Tanner Lectures on Human Values and the opportunity to add this monograph to a prestigious series. I also wish to thank Alan Short for being a generous and thoughtful host when I visited the University of Cambridge to deliver the Tanner Lectures in February of 2022.

Many people guided and stimulated the thinking that culminated in this book. I first began thinking seriously about COVID policy as a participant in an international group of scholars ably led by Ezekiel Emanuel. This work proved valuable preparation for the Tanner Lectures. My views have changed and, I hope, improved a great deal since I presented the Lectures.

Whatever improvements have occurred are due in large part to the generosity of the following people in commenting on my Tanner Lectures or on a series of drafts of this monograph: Jonathan Anomaly, Alex Bird, Cécile Fabre, Elizabeth Levinson, Alexander Motchoulski, Tyler Cowan, and Paul Tucker. I blush to think of the errors and unclarities that these good people helped me to avoid.

I benefited especially from the help of Govind Persad, Robert O. Keohane, and Lance K. Stell. They patiently read and commented on some rather flawed earlier drafts of the lectures and then on drafts of this monograph.

I am also grateful to David Schmidtz, Director of the Center for the Philosophy of Freedom, and to Thomas Christiano, head of the Department of Philosophy, both at the University of Arizona, for their generous support of my research for this volume.

PART I

How to Respond Better to the Next Pandemic
Remedying Institutional Failures

ALLEN BUCHANAN

Delivered at

Clare Hall, University of Cambridge
February 1, 2022

ONE

Policy Failures

There is no shortage of criticisms of governments' responses to COVID-19. Surely, we can respond better to the next pandemic. But how? What lessons for the future can we learn from responses to COVID-19?

Some elements of adequate preparation for the next pandemic are straightforward and uncontroversial. They are commonsense remedies of obvious deficiencies. Examples include more adequate stockpiling of medical supplies, more vigorous efforts to encourage and coordinate vaccine research, improving healthcare infrastructures to function under the stress of a pandemic, developing capacity for vaccine production in less affluent countries, improving early reporting of the emergence of new infectious diseases, and providing more timely, more effective, and better coordinated aid to underresourced countries.

This book makes no attempt to offer a comprehensive set of recommendations for how to prepare for the next pandemic. Instead, its focus is on improving the institutions that shape pandemic policies. My inquiry concentrates on the most important U.S. institutions, the Centers for Disease Control and Prevention (CDC) and the U.S. Department of Health and Human Services (HHS), but much of what I say applies to many other national public health institutions in the United States and abroad. I argue that there was massive institutional failure at the national level, but also with respect to international institutions. I include under the concept of institutional failure the lack of processes and norms that are needed to prevent or reduce the risk of predictable errors and abuses of institutional agents. More positively, sound instutional design requires an aligment of incentives for all actors that can effect outcomes, and alignment that fosters efficient realization of values that policy should serve.

My strategy is preventive. I identify institutional failures that help explain the substantive flaws of COVID-19 pandemic policies and then propose institutional reforms that would reduce the risk of similar institutional failures occurring in the future. I discuss substantive policy errors chiefly to motivate an inquiry into the influence of institutional structures on the policy formation process and the ways in which policies were communicated to the public. My message is that there have been massive institutional failures and that due preparation for the next pandemic requires significant institutional change at the national and international levels. I argue that it is a mistake to locate the ultimate causes of policy failures in poor leadership. Poor leadership was virtually assured, given the flawed institutions within which they made decisions.

SUBSTANTIVE POLICY ERRORS

Here are what I believe to be the most consequential substantive errors in U.S. COVID-19 policy to date.

The Shotgun Strategy

The CDC and the Trump administration opted for a shotgun strategy that inflicted massive economic and psychosocial costs, without evidence that the benefits of this approach would come near to outweighing these costs.[1] So far as I have been able to determine, the chief "evidence" upon which the decision to opt for the shotgun strategy was the word of the Chinese government that it had worked in China! Given that the Chinese government had been far from truthful in the information it provided about the earlier SARS outbreak and taking into account that its pronouncements are not subject to contradiction by domestic actors—due to its ruthless control of the media—relying on this testimony was both

---

1. Maria Nicola et al., "The Socio-economic Implications of the Coronavirus Pandemic (COVID-19): A Review," *International Journal of Surgery* 78 (2020): 185–93; Frederiko Filippini and Eduardo Levi Yeyati, "Pandemic Divergence: The Social and Economic Costs of Covid-19," VoxEU / CEPR, May 12, 2021, https://cepr.org/voxeu/columns/pandemic-divergence -social-and-economic-costs-covid-19; Philip Barrett et al., "After-Effects of the COVID-19 Pandemic: Prospects for Medium-Term Economic Damage," International Monetary Fund Working Papers, July 30, 2021, https://www.imf.org/en/Publications/WP/Issues/2021/07/30 /After-Effects-of-the-COVID-19-Pandemic-Prospects-for-Medium-Term-Economic-Damage -462898—:~:text=While medium-term output losses,size of the policy response.

foolish and irresponsible. When these measures were first considered, the CDC should have heeded available information on their likely serious negative consequences and acknowledged the lack of evidence for their efficacy and then, instead of advocating them, should have forcefully recommended that they not be employed.

Given the high economic and psychosocial costs of the shotgun approach, a better alternative was a targeted strategy that focused on protecting high-risk individuals, namely, those with one or more comorbidities that greatly increase the probability of death or persisting serious negative effects of COVID-19. The use of these high-risk factors did not require testing, so the delay in producing and deploying tests on a large scale cannot excuse the failure to implement a targeted strategy.

Concentrating on reducing exposure of high-risk groups to the virus and prioritizing the treatment of those group members who developed symptoms could have been supplemented by more systematic sampling of municipal wastewater to identify cities that were "hot-spots" (as was the case with New York), in order to channel extra resources to them. Rather than restricting the activities and movement of the majority of the population to prevent them from spreading the virus to the most vulnerable— or on the false assumption that the majority was at serious risk—it would have been more efficient and humane to isolate the most vulnerable and do what could be done to lessen the discomfort and negative psychosocial impact of their isolation. Protecting the most vulnerable by measures that impose great costs and infringements of liberty on the majority was not the best alternative. Or at the very least it required strong evidence not only that it was effective but also that its benefits outweighed the costs and that there was no alternative with a more favorable ratio of benefits to cost. No such evidence was presented to justify the shotgun approach; and none was available.

Here it is worth noting that the adoption of the shotgun approach violated a basic norm governing the adoption of hypotheses that are intended to guide action: if the consequences of proceeding on the assumption that a hypothesis is true are grave should it turn out to be false, then one ought to have exceptionally good evidence in favor of it. To repeat: there was no good evidence that a shotgun approach would produce more benefits than costs much less that there was no less costly but equally effective alternative. And the consequences of acting on the hypothesis that it was effective and efficient were predictably high, should it turn out not to be: massive economic and social harm and serious infringements of liberty

would be inflicted *without compensating benefits*. To say that the requirement of especially strong evidence in favor of the hypothesis was not met
would be a gross understatement.

Vaccine Misinformation

The CDC massively oversold vaccination, conveying the impression that
the new vaccines, like other vaccines with which people were familiar,
would prevent infection and prevent transmission, neither of which was
true.[2] In fact, the chief benefit of the vaccines is that in some, although not
all, cases they reduce the severity of symptoms.

At the time that the safety and efficacy requirements certified by the
Food and Drug Administration (FDA) were satisfied, the CDC knew
that there was no good evidence that the vaccines prevented infection or
transmission. If that was so, then the CDC perpetrated a massive fraud
on the public by implying that one would not become infected and would
not transmit the disease to others if one were vaccinated—conveying the
false message that vaccination was the solution to the COVID-19 problem. Its repeated claim, that by getting vaccinated one was protecting not
only oneself but others, was false: one wasn't protecting others because
the vaccines do not stop transmission; and one wasn't protecting oneself
from becoming infected. Without the disclaimer that, unlike the vaccines the public was most familiar with, these vaccines did not prevent
infection, the "protect yourself" part of the message was bound to be
misinterpreted.

By not making it clear that the vaccines only reduced the severity of
symptoms (in some but not all infected persons) and by not distinguishing these new vaccines from well-known vaccines for measles, mumps,
whooping cough, etc.—which do conclusively prevent infection and
transmission—the CDC provided false assurance to the public. It also
fostered the stigmatization of those who refused vaccination, with disastrous consequences. Such individuals were portrayed as selfishly and irra-
tionally refusing to take a measure that protected not just themselves but
other people to whom they might transmit the disease. Private companies,
medical facilities, and public agencies fired individuals who refused vaccination, unless they were willing to profess a religious objection to vaccination, and unvaccinated athletes were not permitted to enter the country to

2. Marty Makary and Tracy Beth Høeg, "U.S. Public Health Agencies Aren't 'Following
the Science,' Officials Say," *The Free Press*, July 14, 2022, https://www.commonsense.news/p/us
-public-health-agencies-arent-following?s=r&utm_campaign=posset&utm_medium=web.

compete in important events for which they had trained for years. Once it is understood that the vaccines do not prevent infection or transmission, the refusal of some individuals to use a radically new technology is more understandable. And branding them as irrational, fanatical "anti-vaxxers" is shown to be grossly unfair. Given the relative lack of efficacy and the fact that they involved novel mechanisms and were hurried into use, it was not irrational to refuse them, at least if, like the vast majority of Americans, one was not at high risk.

Inadequate Test Kit Planning

The CDC initially took it upon itself to be the sole producer of COVID-19 test kits, in spite of the fact that it lacked experience, expertise, and capacity for test-kit development and production. The initial test kits it produced were defective, due to contamination of some of their components. Correcting this error consumed valuable time. Further, the knowledge that the CDC was developing test kits almost certainly deterred private companies from doing so, out of fear that only CDC kits would be certified by the government or because of the concern that free CDC kits would make selling kits unprofitable. Critics have argued that it would have been much better for the CDC, in cooperation with the FDA, to stimulate and coordinate efforts by major labs to produce test kits.[3]

In addition, the CDC did not exert leadership in addressing a related problem, nor did it urge some other government agency, such as the Department of Health and Human Services (HHS), to do so; even when test kits finally became available in large quantities, there was insufficient capacity for ascertaining and delivering the results. It appears that there was inadequate planning with regard to the capacity and delivery problem, if there was any planning at all.

Misuse of Vaccines for Children

Apparently in response to pressure from the Biden White House, the FDA recently approved and promoted the use of vaccination for infants and children, in spite of the fact that this group is not at high risk and in spite of the fact that there was no evidence that this vaccination would be effective in preventing infection and transmission. There was tremendous pressure on parents to vaccinate their very young children.

---

3. Scott Gottlieb, *Uncontrolled Spread: Why COVID-19 Crushed Us and How We Can Defeat the Next Pandemic* (New York: Harper Collins, 2021), chap. 7.

A number of experts have criticized this policy, expressing the concern that the meager benefits may well be outweighed by the risk of adverse developmental effects on children.[4] In brief, government at the highest levels strongly advocated a vaccination program in the absence of due consideration of risks. That might have been justified if very young children were at significant risk of death or serious persisting negative effects of COVID-19 infection and if there was evidence that the new vaccines would lower this risk, but neither was the case. Neither was the case. The worry of adverse effects in the long-term made large-scale use of the new vaccine all the more dubious.

Here it might be said in defense of the push for vaccinating all infants and young children that it was justified by the successful precedent of the polio vaccination. That vaccine, too, was novel and it was rushed into use. The case of the polio vaccine is strikingly disanalogous, however. The risk of COVID-19 for infants and young children was nothing like the risk of polio—a risk that may well have justified mass administration of the polio vaccine without much evidence of long-term safety. Further, there was evidence that the polio vaccine, in contrast to the COVID-19 vaccine, actually prevented infection.

INSTITUTIONAL FAILURES

In my judgment, the preceding four criticisms are valid and serious. My focus in this volume, however, is not on substantive policy errors but on institutional defects. Once we understand the seriousness of the institutional defects, it will come as no surprise that there were serious substantive errors in policy. That is because the national and international institutional defects I identify not only contributed to bad decision-making *but also reduced the probability that substantive policy errors would be detected and corrected in a timely fashion.* The institutional defects that I list are so serious as to warrant referring to them as institutional failures.

Lack of Public Justifications for Policies

CDC and HHS officials and spokespersons for Presidents Trump and Biden failed to provide anything approaching adequate public justifications for their policies and recommendations, in spite of the fact that they were controversial, even within the relevant scientific communities. At minimum, an adequate public justification would have to include

4. See, for example, *Sensible Medicine* (blog), https://sensiblemed.substack.com/.

(1) a nontechnical presentation of the results of a cost-benefit analysis, showing that the benefits of the policy can reasonably be expected to exceed the costs, and (2) with public access to the analysis itself and to the sources on which the analysis was based.

Showing that the benefits of a proposed policy (significantly) outweigh the costs, where "cost" is construed very broadly and not limited to financial costs, is a minimal requirement for justification. Yet no cost-benefit results were presented to the public for any of the policies the U.S. public health authorities and the executive branch opted for. Instead, the standard procedure was simply to assert or imply, rather than argue, that a policy, if implemented, would produce benefits, with no mention of attendant costs and no effort to show that the recommended policy had a superior ratio of benefits to costs to other less disruptive alternatives.[5] Later, I examine in detail the proper role of cost-benefit analysis in justifying public policies. For now it is enough to say that conducting cost-benefit analysis is a necessary first step in evaluating—and hence in justifying—a policy initiative. If the costs of a policy exceed the benefits, it is a nonstarter.

Nor was the question of *whether the costs would be fairly distributed publicly* broached, much less addressed. This question is extremely important because the policies that the CDC endorsed resulted in dramatically differing costs for different groups—and tended to impose the greatest burdens on people who were already disadvantaged. That was especially true in the case of school closings and lockdowns of "nonessential" businesses. For example, less wealthy parents could ill afford to be absent from work to care for children who were not in school and also were less well-equipped to provide effective home schooling. Further, studies indicate that the negative impact of absence from school on poorer children is much greater than on wealthier ones.[6] In addition, lockdowns of nonessential businesses in the service sector had a disproportionate negative impact on low-wage workers who, unlike the bureaucrats who recommended closing restaurants, bars, cruises, etc., could not work from home. Even if the

5. A notable exception was a CDC-sponsored study that concluded that school closings were not needed because schools were not a major cite of transmission of the COVID virus. However, the CDC embraced the policy of closing schools anyway.

6. Francesco Agostinelli et al., "When the Great Equalizer Shuts Down: Schools, Peers, and Parents in Pandemic Times," *Journal of Public Economics* 206 (2022): 1–10, https://www .sciencedirect.com/science/article/pii/S0047272721002103; Mike Cummings, "COVID school closures most harm students from poorest neighborhoods," *Yale News*, January 5, 2021, https://news.yale.edu/2021/01/05/covid-school-closures-most-harm-students-poorest -neighborhoods.

decentralized nature of the American political system meant that neither the CDC nor the White House could nullify bad decisions made by governments at state and local levels, these two high-level entities were in a unique position to take the lead in foregrounding the point that the distribution of the costs of various strategies should be fair or at least not significantly unfair. They failed to do so.

Just as important, COVID-19 policymakers, from the CDC and HHS to two presidents to local officials, did not take to heart a key tenet of liberal-democratic political orders, first clearly articulated by John Stuart Mill in his classic book *On Liberty*: measures that limit liberty always bear a heavy burden of justification and this burden does not disappear even if we are in a supposed emergency.[7] Discharging that justificatory burden requires making a strong case that there is no less restrictive, less liberty-limiting effective alternative to the policy the government is adopting or recommending. This crucial task was not undertaken, much less successfully performed.

The costs to liberty generally were not even acknowledged by policymakers; and this sent a message to the public that infringement of their liberty did not matter to those in power. Unsurprisingly, on the Right, the government's apparent callous disregard of liberty spawned a conspiracy theory that COVID-related restrictions were designed to prime the public to accept greater limitations on liberty, undertaken for more sinister reasons, in the future. My surmise is that this failure to acknowledge the gravity of infringements of liberty contributed to the legitimacy deficit that public health authorities accrued during the pandemic. The point is not that infringement of liberty is never justified; it is that the seriousness of liberty infringement ought to be publicly acknowledged. And the impact on liberty should count as a significant cost in any cost-benefit analysis.[8]

Failure to Take Dissenting Views Seriously

Pandemic policymakers in the United States did not make a sincere effort, if they made any effort at all, to solicit and respond on the merits to reasonable criticisms of their strategies, before or after enacting them. There is no evidence that the process of policy formulation included effective measures to ensure that the public health national leadership's views received serious critical scrutiny. Nor has there been a public announcement by the top public health authorities promising either periodic critical reviews of

7. John Stuart Mill, *On Liberty* (Indianapolis: Hackett Publishing, 1978), chap. V.

8. Jonny Anomaly, "Public Health and Public Goods," *Public Health Ethics* 4, no. 3 (2011): 251–59.

policy during the pandemic nor a post-hoc review after the pandemic is declared officially over.

Even worse, in at least one prominent case, instead of acknowledging that there was reasonable disagreement, the director of the HHS, Francis Collins, in an email to Anthony Fauci, director of the Infectious Diseases section of the CDC, urged a policy of discrediting critics of the official policy, including the highly respected authors of the Great Barrington Declaration, branding them as quacks and eccentrics, rather than engaging with them on the issues.[9] More generally, there was a notable failure to acknowledge publicly and respond on the merits to credible dissenting voices.

I have found no evidence of a serious effort to articulate or give voice to dissenting views in the internal workings of the CDC, HHS, or the FDA. In other words, during the process of formulating policy, there was no institutional mechanism that was the equivalent of an official devil's advocate position to challenge the official view and no effective requirement of responding to such a dissenting view if it were voiced. If, contrary to what we know, there were due consideration of dissenting voices in the process of policy formulation, this was not made public; as a result, the public was deprived of the assurance that the policies adopted were well-considered and the opportunity to question whether the dissenting views may have been correct and whether government responses to them were adequate.

Given the tendency of subordinates to say what their powerful superiors want to hear, the lack of such a mechanism, and more generally the absence of an institutional commitment to taking criticisms seriously, almost certainly contributed to the "yes men" and "group think" phenomena that are common in large-scale institutions that wield significant power. To assume that public health workers are immune to this ubiquitous pathology of organizations is to assume, without warrant, that they are radically different from the rest of humanity simply because they are in the public sector. Such an idealization is as dangerous as it is naïve.

Misrepresentation of the Nature and Scope of Expertise

CDC and HHS officials, as well as state and local public health authorities, *failed to make clear to the public the limits and nature of public health*

---

9. In an email to Anthony Fauci, Director of the Infectious Diseases section of the CDC, Francis Collins urged a policy of discrediting critics of the CDC's official policy. See "How Fauci and Collins Shut Down Covid Debate" by the Editorial Board at *The Wall Street Journal,* https://www.wsj.com/articles/fauci-collins-emails-great-barrington-declaration-covid-pandemic-lockdown-11640129116.

expertise. In doing so they foisted on the public a profound misunderstanding of their roles and the proper mission of their agencies. Even worse, they actively misrepresented their expertise. Every major policy decision was in fact a conclusion based not just on scientific premises but also on moral assumptions, in particular assumptions about how to make proper trade-offs when there are conflicts among values. And these assumptions were usually controversial, far from self-evidently true. For example, it was simply assumed, at least implicitly, that the massive economic and psychosocial costs of lockdowns and school closings—and their unequal distribution—was justified by the supposed gains in slowing (not stopping) the spread of the virus. Or, less charitably, policymakers did not first acknowledge that these costs mattered and then go on to make the case that they were acceptable in order to reap the supposed benefits. Instead, they focused only on *supposed* benefits or, more accurately, on one supposed benefit, namely, the reduction of harm from the virus. Rather than acknowledging that their policy choices were based in part on moral judgments about proper trade-offs among conflicting values, these officials gave the impression that they were based solely on scientific expertise.

To my knowledge, the only justification for making slowing the spread of the virus an overriding goal was to avoid overloading the medical system. One wonders, however, whether the best way to protect the medical system from overload was to employ such costly, distributively unfair, and disruptive policies. Instead, perhaps more could have been done to strengthen the medical system's capacity, for example, by accelerating graduation of nurses and doctors, easing immigration restrictions on medical personnel, and more fully utilizing medical personnel from the armed forces, where this would include mobilizing reserves and extending tours of duty. Another alternative would have been a mixed strategy: less draconian lockdowns combined with various strategies for augmenting medical capacity.

Of course, the targeted strategy takes more time to implement, so the case could be made that the extremely costly shotgun approach was warranted in an emergency. The problem with this reply is twofold: first, it is not clear that overloading the medical system would have been as harmful as the shotgun approach; but second, at most this would justify much shorter lockdowns and school closings than were in fact implemented, to gain time for implementing more targeted strategies.

It is important to understand that the threat of overload was not ubiquitous; some cities and counties were vulnerable, others were not.

Consequently, a more targeted strategy, focusing on enhancing capacity where it was weak, might well have had a higher ratio of benefits to costs. Simply to assume that the negative effects of overloading the medical system would be greater than the negative effects of lockdowns and school closings, without doing the cost-benefit analysis, is irrational. Given the harms of such drastic interventions, it is also morally irresponsible. A better approach would have considered the possibility that some negative effects of stress on medical services was a reasonable price to pay if the alternative was much greater human damage due to draconian lockdown policies.

My point is not that it is obvious what the proper trade-off was; rather, it is that such trade-offs must be carefully considered, but apparently were not. If, as seems very unlikely, there was serious reasoning concerning trade-offs in the internal workings of the CDC, that would not suffice. The public is owed a justification for controversial, costly, and liberty-limiting policies; and justification requires an explicit account of how trade-offs were handled.

Just as important, officials at every level, from the CDC and HHS down to mayors and school boards, *misrepresented* the nature of science. They neglected to convey to the public the fact that there was significant and reasonable disagreement among genuine experts as to the supposed scientific facts upon which they based their policies. Instead, they promulgated a distorted understanding of what science is. By falsely conveying the impression that science spoke with one voice (theirs), officials positioned themselves to charge anyone who disagreed with them as refusing to "follow the science." This convenient lie foreclosed rational discussion of policy alternatives, which in turn reduced the quality of the decision-making process and hindered early detection and correction of policy errors.

In addition, there was a tendency to convey greater certainty about the facts and the efficacy of recommended policies than was warranted. For example, in the absence of a surveillance system that included mass testing, the CDC initially announced that it was adequately prepared to handle the COVID-19 virus and provided unfounded assurances that the virus was not a major threat in the United States.[10] The point is that in the absence of mass testing data, both the claim that the CDC was prepared and the assurance that the virus posed no major threat were unfounded in the early

---

10. Sarah Owemohle and Adam Cancryn, "Top Health Officials Warn Senators More Wuhan Virus Cases Likely," *Politico*, January 24, 2020, https://www.politico.com/news/2020/01/24/coronavirus-united-states-103580.

context of uncertainty as to how serious the disease was. Manipulative recourse to misinformation, along with excessive claims of certainty and false assurances, in the end backfired, contributing to a loss of credibility on the part of the CDC and HHS that will make a sound response to the next pandemic more difficult if not impossible.[11]

Wrongful Political Influence on Policy

Pandemic policy at the highest national levels was subject to *wrongful political influence*. In two prominent cases, the influence came from the Executive Branch. President Trump pressured the FDA director to grant Emergency Use Authorization to the drug hydroxychloroquine, a compound that studies showed to be inefficacious in treating COVID-19 and to have serious side effects. More recently, as noted earlier, the Biden White House pressured the CDC to recommend vaccination for very young children, in spite of the fact that studies by the vaccine makers themselves indicated that there was very little benefit, and in the absence of data on long-term developmental effects of administering vaccines to this population. The institutional failure in this case is the absence of firewalls, legal barriers between elected officials, and above all the executive branch, and the agencies tasked with responding to a pandemic. Measures to reduce the risk of interference by elected officials have been successfully adopted in other countries, including Sweden.[12] Yet in the United States there has not even been a public debate concerning the need for them.

International Institutional Failure: Inadequate and Uncoordinated Aid to Less Wealthy Countries

There was also institutional failure at the *international level*. Although both the governments of well-resourced countries and the pharmaceutical companies producing vaccines publicly acknowledged that they ought to "do something" to aid countries who lacked the resources to cope effectively with the pandemic, aid was inadequate and uncoordinated. The idea that there was a duty to render aid was left indeterminate as to the duty's content and extent, with the predictable result that there was serious

11. Gottlieb, *Uncontrolled Spread*, 75: "The United States would never deploy enough tests to implement widespread screening, even for a rudimentary surveillance effort. In the absence of surveillance testing, health officials were forced to rely largely on a far les ssensitive tool to tell whether corona virus was starting to spread in local communities: syndromic surveillance."

12. Lars Jonung, "Sweden's Constitution Decides Its Exceptional Covid-19 Policy," *VoxEU*, June 18, 2020, https://cepr.org/voxeu/columns/swedens-constitution-decides-its-exceptional-covid-19-policy.

moral under-performance. Several international organizations endeavored to make vaccines more affordable for poorer countries, but their efforts were both largely ineffective and subject to criticisms on grounds of inequity and lack of transparency. Wealthy countries amassed amounts of vaccines far in excess of their needs and did not distribute surpluses to needy countries.[13]

THE PLAN OF THIS BOOK

The first three national institutional failures listed above are presented in what I take to be the order of their importance. The coming chapters exhibit a different ordering, one that is designed to motivate the work of the two constructive chapters, Four and Five, in which I propose national and international institutional reforms respectively. Chapter Six, on the destructive influence of public health ideology, is admittedly more speculative than the rest.

Chapter Two develops in detail the third institutional failure, the misrepresentation of the nature of public health expertise and of the nature of science. There I explain why there is an unavoidable nonscientific moral element in policy decisions. I note several different trade-offs that pandemic policies reflected, and demonstrate that they cannot be determined by scientific reasoning. "Trade-offs" here means judgments that balance conflicting goals or values or in extreme cases assign absolute precedence to one value when it conflicts with others.

I then show that public health experts as such have no expertise in making trade-offs. Often, they proceed as if it were not necessary to make trade-offs, because policy decisions are determined by "the science," or they assume that their expertise as public health professionals gives them the authority to make trade-offs. Then I show how economic expertise, although it may be necessary for making reasonable trade-offs, is not sufficient to do so and that the belief that it is on the part of some economists is the result either of the false assumption that a single-minded pursuit of efficiency is "morally neutral" or the unsupported assumption that utilitarianism is the correct moral view. The former assumption is patently false; the latter is hotly disputed throughout the history of moral philosophy up to the present day.

13. G. Owen Schaefer, R. J. Leland, and Ezekiel Emaneul, "Making Vaccines Available to Other Countries Before Offering Domestic Booster Vaccinations," *JAMA* 326, no. 10 (2021): 902–4; Talha Burki, "Global COVID-19 Vaccine Inequity," *The Lancet Infectious Disesases* 21, no. 7 (2021): 922–23.

In assuming that trade-offs are to be governed solely by the criterion of efficiency, economists are grossly overselling their own expertise. They either are mistakenly assuming that efficiency in the technical economic sense is all that matters in making trade-offs, thereby overlooking the fact that efficient outcomes can be unjust or otherwise morally deficient; or they are arbitrarily assuming the validity of an especially controversial moral theory, namely, utilitarianism, and using efficiency as a proxy for what maximizes overall utility. It is one thing to invoke a moral theory; quite another to do so without making any effort to defend it against well-known criticisms while pretending that one is doing strictly scientific economic analysis.

I also show how failure to acknowledge the nature and limits of science contributed to misguided controversies about COVID-19 policy and obscured the roots of policy deficiencies. Two misrepresentations are especially damaging: pretending that science speaks with one voice on matters relevant to pandemic response policies; and presenting scientific views with greater certainty than is warranted. One effect of this combination of misrepresentations is to deflect criticism of policies by accusing those who oppose them as refusing "to follow the science."

Chapter Three explores the fourth institutional failure, undue political influence in the broader context of pandemic politics. I define "politics" as most political scientists do: as the struggle for power—for getting it, holding on to it, and constraining or displacing those who possess it. I focus on three domains of politics: (1) the internal politics of the top-level public health agencies charged with leading the response to the pandemic; (2) political influence on these agencies coming from forces outside them, especially from the executive branch of the U.S. Federal Government; and (3) the politicization of the public debate about and reaction to government COVID-19 policy that resulted from the current polarized, indeed tribalistic character of American society.

In considering the first domain, the internal politics of the highest-level public health agencies, I rely on two points, both of which enjoy a broad consensus in political science and organization theory. The first is that hierarchical organizations suppress dissent or make it costly. The second is that the "group think" or "yes men" phenomenon is present in public as well as private organizations. In addition, my analysis takes seriously the fact that public health experts, like experts generally, have a strong incentive to overestimate both the extent and the depth of their expertise, by which their power and prestige is thereby enhanced. I also emphasize another fact about experts, including public health experts: the fact that a person has chosen to invest much time and effort into acquiring certain skills generally reflects an overly generous estimate of how important those skills are. (Hence the old saying: if one has a hammer, especially if one has invested a lot in getting the hammer, everything looks like a nail.) This too can lead to a failure to recognize the limits of one's expertise, which in turn can undercut the effectiveness of even the best-intentioned action.

With respect to the second domain of pandemic politics, political influence on public health policymakers coming from external agents, I have already noted that the Biden White House apparently pressured the FDA to approve the use of vaccines in very young children, without good evidence of significant efficacy and that this was a dubious decision, given that there was a possibility of serious long-term adverse effects of applying this new technology to individuals at an early stage of their development. I also point out that President Trump wrongly pressured the FDA to certify Emergency Authorization Use status for of hydroxychloroquine, a drug that turned out to be ineffective against COVID-19 and unsafe as well.

The bulk of my discussion of pandemic politics, however, is devoted to the third domain, exploring the role of politics in the larger environment in which pandemic policy was forged. I focus on the impact of the extreme affective polarization—or, as I prefer to term it, tribalism—that afflicts American life today. Tribalism is distinct from and more destructive than polarization. To say that there is polarization means simply that there are large substantive differences on policy issues and that they are growing. Polarization is compatible with rational discussion and with opposing groups respecting each other. Tribalism is not. When the tribalistic mentality takes hold all issues are bundled together in a supposed supreme emergency, a no-holds-barred, zero-sum struggle for the highest stakes; and the Other is regarded as incapable of being reasoned with, either because they are irremediably stupid or misinformed or because they are irredeemably corrupt and insincere. Discourse becomes a matter of sorting and signaling—sorting people into Us versus Them and signaling total allegiance to our side. There is no engagement on the substantive issues and no possibility of bargaining and compromise, because the Other is denied the status of a being we can reason with and because it is assumed that all conflicts are zero sum, with no possibility of meeting in the middle. Because bargaining and compromise are essential for democracy to work, tribalism destroys democracy.

My chief point is that tribalism is a formidable obstacle to reasonable public discussion of pandemic policy and, in addition, deprives public health leaders of the legitimacy they must have if their policies are to be effective. By "legitimacy" here I mean perceived rightful authority. Without legitimacy, compliance with policies that require curbing self-interest can only be made effective, if it can be made effective at all, by excessive coercion.[14]

In Chapter Four, I address remedies for the first national institutional failure, the lack of adequate public justifications for pandemic policies as an element of a more comprehensive set of proposed institutional changes designed to improve the decision-making processes of the national institutions chiefly responsible for pandemic policy. The overarching aim of these recommendations is to make the decision-makers accountable, first and foremost by requiring them to provide public justifications for their decisions, where this includes not only the public presentation of the results of cost-benefit analyses but also positive efforts to elicit and reply responsibly to dissenting views; and second, to ensure that policy proposals are seriously questioned prior to making the public case for them. I also propose mandatory periodic impartial reviews of official behavior.

Accountability requires (1) a standard for evaluating behavior, (2) an accountability-holder, some agent or agents tasked with determining whether actors' behavior satisfies the standards, and (3) some mechanism for imposing significant costs on actors whose behavior fails to satisfy the standard. Broad accountability features, in addition (4), some effective provision for reevaluating the terms of accountability over time, where this includes critical appraisal of the standards, the choice of accountability holders, and the costs for bad performance.[15]

Whether any institution can achieve legitimacy under current conditions of tribalism is not obvious. The worst effect of tribalism is that policies are not evaluated on their merits: instead, the first question is "Do They want us to accept that policy?" Will that policy further Their (pernicious) values. Once the messenger is identified as one of Them, the message is rejected. If They attack a policy supported by those We see as on Our side, We must commit to it all the more fully. If one questions a

14. Allen Buchanan and Robert O. Keohane, "The Legitimacy of Global Governance Institutions," *Ethics & International Affairs* 20, no. 4 (2006): 405–37. See also Allen Buchanan, "Institutional Legitimacy," in *Oxford Studies in Political Philosophy Volume 4*, ed. David Sobel, Peter Vellentyne, and Steven Wall (New York: Oxford University Press, 2018), 53–78.

15. Buchanan and Keohane, "The Legitimacy of Global Governance Institutions." None of these elements are present in the case of institutions trusted to deal with the pandemic.

policy that has the stamp of approval of those we regard as representing Our tribe, one runs the risk of being branded a traitor. If tribalism is severe enough, the best of accountability mechanisms may not work: a negative evaluation on institutional performance, no matter how impartially conducted, may be rejected as "rigged," just as the fairest election may be. My claim is only that the institutional reforms I recommend are necessary, not sufficient, for legitimacy—and that legitimacy is necessary for a sound response to the next pandemic.

Chapter Five shifts from national to international institutional reform. I first note that better-resourced countries and medical supply companies, including vaccine makers, while acknowledging that they should do something to help poorer countries cope with the pandemic, failed to do enough and that efforts to distribute vaccines to countries that could not afford them were uncoordinated and of limited effectiveness. I then argue that these shortcomings were the predictable result of framing the duty to aid poorer countries as a duty of charity or beneficence, what moral philosophers call an imperfect duty. If a duty is imperfect, then it is not owed to any specific individuals and the duty-bearer has discretion as to whom to help, how to help them, and when to help them.

Imperfect duties are tailor-made for procrastination, backsliding, and moral underperformance. I argue that properly designed institutions can "perfect" imperfect duties and avoid these shortcomings by clearly specifying duty-bearers and those to whom the duties are owed, fairly distributing the costs of providing help, providing effective mechanisms for compliance with the specified duties that solve the free-rider problem, and providing wealthy countries with assurance that others will do their part in addressing the needs of the less wealthy.

Chapter Six speculates on the role of a certain strand of public health ideology in fostering the uncritical, underevidenced acceptance of the untargeted shotgun policies adopted in the United States and many other countries in response to COVID-19. The framing assumption here is that an ideology can be an element of an institution or at least can shape how an institution functions, and that a flawed ideology can contribute to institutional failures.

I hypothesize that support for the shotgun approach, and the correlative failure to seriously consider more targeted policies, was due in part to a public ideology that includes two elements: (1) the presumption that if there is a public health emergency, measures should be directed toward everyone in a country, everyone subject to the jurisdiction of national public health officials; and (2) the presumption that *the* proper goal of public health measures in a pandemic is to stop the spread of the disease or to reduce as much as possible the health damage due to the disease, without serious consideration of the costs—especially the costs that are not directly related to health—of the pursuit of that goal. The first element precludes strategies that segment the general population into high- and low-risk groups with different policies for each, while the second fosters an irrational preoccupation with only one type of harm, ignoring the negative impact that a single-minded preoccupation with the health effects of a pandemic has on other important values.

My conjecture is that presumption (1) is a hangover from the time at which public health first became a self-conscious profession: when public health measures were not focused on subpopulations, but instead on the public at large, such as improvements in food and water sanitation that prevented diseases that affected virtually everyone. With respect to these sorts of interventions, it made sense to think of public health as dealing with whole populations. And given that effective public health authorities existed only at the national level, that meant whole national populations. Presumption (2) is most likely the result of one instance of a more widespread phenomenon: the tunnel vision of experts. Public health officials are trained to focus primarily on the health effects of infectious diseases; they are not trained as moral philosophers or as economists, both of whom are keenly attentive to trade-offs and to the fact that freedom from infection is not the only worthwhile goal in life. More generally, health care professionals, not just public health experts, have a tendency to reason as if health or freedom from disease were the only good or obviously the most important, which it most clearly is not. They seem to forget that every day, each of us willingly and quite appropriately engages in behavior that is not optimal from a health standpoint, because we are making trade-offs, acknowledging that in some cases the opportunity costs of a strict pursuit of optimal health are too high. That is the case, for example, when we work long hours for a cause we think is of great moral importance or to earn sufficient funds to send our children to a good university.

METHODOLOGY

My approach in this volume, which includes some of my previous work, differs sharply from that of most moral philosophers writing on the current pandemic. The standard strategy is to propose what are thought to be better policies, explaining why they are superior to those actually adopted.

In addition, there has been special emphasis on issues of rationing medical supplies, including vaccines, both within countries and across them.

I have two serious worries about this approach. First of all, the proposals for better policies typically are free floating and disembodied—formulated without any reference to institutional realities or to the actual incentives of those who are supposed to implement them. Little if any attention is paid to the question of whether these agents would be likely to adopt the policies, given their incentives. Free-floating or disembodied approaches are most charitably understood as arguments directed toward ideal agents— agents whose decisions are determined solely by reason and their commitment to doing the right thing—but who are, therefore, quite different from the flesh and blood creatures who actually determine pandemic policies.

Second, no explanation is provided of why less desirable policies have in fact been adopted. Yet one would think that knowing why things have gone wrong would be helpful for knowing how to make them go right in the future. These two worries are related: without any explanation of why institutional agents have opted for what is arguable a morally deficient policy, one has no good reason to think they will adopt the supposedly superior policy the philosopher is recommending. In effect, when the ideal agent perspective is taken, the philosopher seems to be simply counting on the motivational power of sound arguments—if she is assuming that her work is likely to have any practical effect at all.

This tendency to provide free-floating, disembodied arguments—arguments that make no reference to institutional context or the incentives of the agents who are supposed to act on their conclusions—is pervasive in contemporary moral philosophy. A prominent example is contemporary just war theory, which has undergone a dramatic revitalization in the past two decades. The most influential figures in this field describe their work as "pure moral theory."[16] The obvious worry is that, although this work is commendably creative and rigorous, it is unlikely to have any effect whatsoever on war-making for the simple reason that it does not engage the beliefs and motivations of military and civilian leaders.

For one thing, the arguments these theorists provide are so complex and cognitively demanding that few if any who are not trained in moral philosophy will be able follow them, much less be convinced by them. Second, and more importantly, it would be extremely naïve—to subscribe

---

16. See Jeff McMahan, *Killing in War* (Oxford: Clarendon Press, 2009); Jeff McMahan, "The Ethics of Killing in War," *Ethics* 114, no. 4 (2004): 693–733; and Thomas Hurka, "Proportionality in the Morality of War," *Philosophy and Public Affairs* 33, no. 1 (2005): 34–66.

to an extraordinarily dubious rationalist moral psychology—to think that leaders in our world determine their conduct by impartial reasons presented in sound arguments, that they are not instead influenced by incentives that are often orthogonal to the pursuit of moral truth. In brief, pure moral theory may be (trivially) the right theory for pure moral agents, but taken by itself it seems to be of little use in a world in which decisions regarding war are made by radically different sorts of beings.

Some just war theorists acknowledge that this is so and they express the desire that some other (presumably less deep) thinkers undertake the task of showing how their theories could guide proposals for feasible changes in war-making in our world. In other words, they distinguish sharply between ideal (or pure) moral theory and nonideal moral theory and admit that they have only provided the former. The idea is that ideal moral theory sets the moral goal, while nonideal theory tells us how to get there from here. The problem is that, so far at least, the only theories worthy of the name are ideal. In other words, theories that show just how ideal theory can guide feasible reforms regarding the initiation and conduct of war are not at present available. There are some ad hoc and unsystematic attempts to provide reason-supported recommendations for particular institutional reforms regarding war-making, but these tend to rely on widely accepted moral principles rather than on any of the rival ideal just war theories.[17] Consequently, they do not establish the practical value of ideal theory. Without developed nonideal theories, the check issued in the form of an ideal theory cannot be cashed.

The alternative that I favor and have developed in extensive writings on just war issues, and which I pursue in this book, is to begin, not with pure moral theory, but with where we actually are. The idea is to focus on the actual deficiencies of current institutions as these are identified by relatively uncontroversial moral principles available to a range of ideal theories, and then suggest feasible institutional improvements.[18]

Of course, to identify something as a deficiency requires an evaluative perspective. My hope, however, is that the evaluations of institutional performance I make in this book and which provide the impetus for a consideration of institutional reforms are so uncontroversial and indeed

17. Allen Buchanan and Robert O. Keohane, "Precommitment Regimes for Intervention: Supplementing the Security Council," *Ethics and International Affairs* 25, no. 1 (2011): 41–63; Allen Buchanan and Robert O. Keohane, "The Preventative Use of Force: A Cosmopolitan Institutional Proposal," *Ethics and International Affairs* 18, no. 1 (2004): 1–22.

18. Allen Buchanan, *Institutionalizing the Just War* (New York: Oxford University Press, 2018).

commonsensical that they do not require a deep moral theory. To put the same point most simply: in some contexts, one can make some moral assumptions—without producing a bulletproof cognitivist metaethical theory and without showing that the assumption can be derived from some rock-bottom ethical principle or small set of principles. The basic idea of my approach is to begin with where we are, not with where we ought, ideally, to be.

I cheerfully acknowledge that there is a place for foundational, deep moral theorizing. I simply deny that the current volume is the place. To proceed, as I do, on the assumption that officials in a democratic polity owe citizens a public justification for policies that significantly limit liberty and impose unequally distributed economic and psychosocial costs does not require a deep normative theory much less a metaethical view capable of refuting moral nihilists. For one thing, it is pretty clear that the failure to bear the burden of public justification, along with the near total absence of post hoc accountability for policy choices, is a recipe for bad decisions. We know enough about human beings to be confident that power without accountability is dangerous, subject both to honest errors and to abuse. Nonetheless, in Chapter Four, I argue that the public justification requirement is not just of instrumental value, a tool for avoiding bad consequences: it is also supported by an appealing and widely influential philosophical theory, justificatory liberalism, according to which coercive institutions are legitimate only if they can be justified to all over whom they exercise authority. More basically, public justification is required by equal respect for persons, whether justificatory liberalism is the correct moral-political theory or not.

The key point is that how deep into moral theory one needs to go depends upon what one's aims are and whom one is addressing. My aim is to provide resources for a better response to the next pandemic; it is not to convince anyone that what I say can be deduced from some foundational comprehensive moral theory that answers all the questions normative ethical theorists and metaethicists have the leisure (and freedom from the responsibility that goes with making practical suggestions) to pursue.[19]

An advantage of my approach is that it is more likely to have some practical impact than the pure moral theory or disembodied argument

19. Normative ethical theorizing takes as its subject the content of moral judgments, attempting to delineate moral standards that provide us with norms or standards for ethical behavior. Metaethics is the examination of the nature and limitations of morality. Rather than asking what morality demands of us, metaethics asks what morality is.

approach. Its focus is on how institutions could be improved. It does not rely on officials being persuaded by abstract argument. Instead, it relies on the fact that agents respond to the incentives that institutions create.

Of course, there is the question of whether those with the power to do so will enact the institutional reforms I recommend. In Chapter Four, when I set out the institutional changes needed to improve decision-making at the national level, I begin—but only begin—to make the case that what I recommend is feasible. The key point here is that the institutional mechanisms for accountability I propose are far from novel, having already been adopted in some quarters of governance, and that they *are so commonsensical as to garner widespread popular support, support capable of pressuring those in power to adopt them*. Most importantly, the U.S. domestic reforms I propose would not be initiated by those subject to them: instead, they would be enacted by Congress. So, I am not expecting those in need of being held accountable to make themselves accountable. I am depending on the fact that in the United States and other liberal-democratic constitutional orders, bureaucrats are answerable to the legislative branch and ultimately to the legislative. I am also assuming that there has been such a loss of credibility on the part of the top public health bureaucracies as a result of their actions during the COVID-19 pandemic, that there would be popular support for institutional reform. My hope is that if a clear program of reform were presented and publicly justified, key civil society groups could mobilize public pressure on Congress to enact it.

"THE NEXT" PANDEMIC

It is helpful to distinguish two quite different scenarios. In the first, there is no end for the COVID-19 pandemic, or rather the pandemic becomes endemic (this may already have occurred). We come to talk of "COVID season" in the way we have spoken of flu season. The infection never dies out, rather it subsides and then flares up periodically, especially in the Fall and Winter. If we are lucky, the case mortality rate declines. COVID becomes—for most but not all of us—merely a once yearly inconvenience. Some people still die of COVID; but the same is true of the flu.

The second scenario is different, and more worrisome. There are two versions. According to the first, the COVID-19 virus (or rather some current variant) significantly mutates so that we return to a situation like that of March 2020: there is a genuine pandemic, an acute health crisis. Alternatively, a new virus, not a variant of COVID-19, erupts.

When I speak of preparing for the next pandemic, I have the second scenario in mind, not the case of endemic disease. Yet if the institutional reforms I recommend were implemented, they would improve public health decision-making at the top, whether in response to the first or the second scenario.

TWO

The Misrepresentation of Expertise

In Chapter One, I observed that experts generally, and not just public health experts, have strong incentives to oversell their expertise, both with respect to its breadth (which matters fall within their expertise) and with respect to its depth (how good their knowledge is regarding those matters that fall within their expertise). Both sorts of misrepresentations, if accepted by the public, enhance the experts' power and prestige and usually their financial condition as well. A classic instance of the misrepresentation of expertise is well-documented in the literature on medical paternalism.[1] Although there have been some improvements in recent years, physicians have traditionally misrepresented the scope of their expertise, often making morally controversial decisions regarding the use or withdrawing of life support while presenting them as being medical decisions.

Here are two examples among many. During the 1970s, physicians in the UK routinely denied access to dialysis to patients over sixty-five.[2] But instead of admitting that this was a morally controversial rationing policy, they told their patients that dialysis was "not suitable" or "not indicated"

1. Allen Buchanan, "Medical Paternalism," *Philosophy & Public Affairs* 7, no. 4 (1978): 370–90.

2. Jennifer Stanton, "The Cost of Living: Kidney Dialysis, Rationing and Health Economics in Britain, 1965–1996," *Social Science & Medicine* 49, no. 9 (1999): 1169–82; Roberta G. Simmons and Susan Klein Marine, "The Regulation of High Cost Technology Medicine: The Case of Dialysis and Transplantation in the United Kingdom," *Journal of Health and Social Behavior* 25, no. 3 (1984): 320–34.

for them.[3] Similarly, at least through the 1960s, American physicians often refused to undertake life-saving surgeries and organ transplants on Down Syndrome babies, without offering parents the opportunity to participate in a consideration of options, and justified this behavior by saying that they were better qualified to make the decision than the parents. In some cases, like British physicians denying access to dialysis, they disguised the fact that they were making controversial moral judgments for which they had no training by saying that surgery wasn't indicated for babies like this.[4] In other cases, they simply assumed that the quality of life of a Down Syndrome individual was so low that death would be superior to life. In effect, they assumed that the proper role of the physician was to make morally controversial judgments about the value of impaired newborns' lives. Yet nothing in the domain of their expertise, nothing in their training, qualified them to serve as experts on the value of lives. These physicians acted as if they were moral experts, but pretended they were merely exercising their medical expertise.

WHY EXPERTS TEND TO EXAGGERATE
THE DEPTH AND BREADTH OF THEIR EXPERTISE

In addition to enhancing the expert's power and prestige, a successful claim that some matter falls within their expertise also has the effect of disabling potential criticism of the expert's behavior or judgments. If someone challenges her, an expert will reply that the challenger both fails to acknowledge genuine expertise and falsely claims to be an expert. This function of expertise is most effective if one can convince people not just that one is an expert but that one is the only, or best qualified, expert.

When an institution is created to exercise authority in a particular domain, as was the case with the CDC, and it is recognized as the highest authority in that domain, it becomes much easier for its agents to make a credible claim that they are the sole authorities or the most qualified experts in that domain. The effect is to make it much harder for anyone outside the institution to question the institutional agents' claims to superior knowledge. Given that this is so, it is all the more important to devise specific institutional mechanisms to empower dissenting voices. It is of at

3. "Audit in Renal Failure: The Wrong Target?" *British Medical Journal* 283, no. 6286 (1981): 261–62.

4. Elizabeth Cohen, "Disabled Baby Denied Heart Transplant," CNN Health, November 30, 2013. https://www.cnn.com/2013/11/30/health/disabled-transplants. See also John M. Maciejczyk, "Withholding Treatment from Defective Infants: Infant Doe Postmortem," *Notre Dame Law Review* 59, no.1 (1983): 224–52.

least equal importance for the public to be clear about the nature and limitations of the expertise that institutional agents claim to possess. Unless this is done, dissenting voices will be facilely dismissed as unqualified.

The first major—and unacknowledged—limitation on the expertise of the agents authorized to take the lead in pandemic policy is that they do not possess a monopoly on scientific truth. There is seldom complete agreement among scientists on the facts. Indeed, science progresses through vigorous disagreement. Spokespersons for the CDC, HHS, and two presidents have not acknowledged the existence of scientific disagreements and have instead given the impression that those who disagree with their policies are rejecting science. Such a posture to head off what might in fact be valid criticisms is not only dishonest and contrived but also self-defeating in that when the official "facts" turn out to be false, there is a well-deserved loss of credibility.

Here it is important to emphasize that the subterfuge of claiming to possess "the scientific truth" is wholly predictable. Officials have strong incentives to adopt it. Doing so shields them from criticism, allowing them to brand those who disagree as "anti-science" or "refusing to follow the science."

There are two distinct facts about science that must be repeatedly conveyed to the public in official communications regarding pandemic policy. The first, which I have already noted, is that science does not speak with one voice in most instances; the second is that even when it does, it should not project certainty but rather humility, a recognition that even the best science is fallible. The message should be an admission of fallibility along, with a clear statement of the fact that although science doesn't always get it right, it tends to get things "righter"; that is, science is better than other ways of knowing at detecting and correcting its mistakes.

It may well be that government officials, including those working in highest level public health authorities, generally tend to exaggerate the certainty of their views and the extent of scientific consensus they enjoy out of fear that doing otherwise will lead people to question their expertise and hence limit their power and freedom of action. If that is so, then it is remarkably shortsighted, because a greater loss of credibility is bound to occur when their supposed certainties turn out to be mistaken. This phenomenon recurred with disturbing regularity in the case of CDC communications during the COVID-19 pandemic. First we were told that contaminated objects, or fomites, were the big problem; then it turned out they weren't. Next we were told masks weren't effective, then that they were. Then we were told that vaccination would prevent reinfection; then it was admitted that it does not. Correction of mistaken views need not undermine credibility; but correction of views that were presented as certain does.

To summarize: institutional agents have strong incentives to misrepresent their expertise because doing so both enhances their power and prestige and insulates them from valid challenges to their policies in the short-run. Yet in the longer run, such misrepresentation makes them vulnerable to losing the credibility they must have to do their job. Because there are strong incentives for public health officials to misrepresent the scope and depth of their expertise and to exaggerate the degree of scientific support for their strategies, it is necessary to devise effective counter-incentives. Unless this is done, public health officials will continue to destroy what is perhaps the most crucial resource for responding effectively to the next pandemic: their credibility.

A point made earlier bears emphasis: when experts misrepresent the breadth or depth of their expertise, the problem is not just that they are deceiving the public and garnering authority, power, and prestige to which they have no right, though that is bad enough. Even worse, they are disabling valid criticism of what they do by discrediting those who challenge them, branding critics as inferior sources of knowledge and as benighted people who obstinately fail to recognize the valid claims of expertise. *By impugning the standing of those who attempt to hold experts accountable, the misrepresentation of expertise facilitates bad decision-making while making detection and correction of errors all the more difficult.* When someone questions their actions, the experts reply: "You are not in a position to say that; if you knew what we know, you would approve our actions; but you can't know that because you lack our expertise." Note that this strategy of discrediting the challenger conveniently avoids having to respond to the substance of the challenge: the message is disregarded by denying the messenger's standing. Yet being required to respond to critics on the substance is often necessary for detecting and correcting mistakes.

LIBERAL BIAS AMONG SCIENTISTS?

So far, I have emphasized the dangers of exaggerated claims of expertise; but there is another risk, namely, that people will fail to recognize genuine expertise with the result that policy choices are not properly guided by expertise. This can occur if people believe that scientists, including public health experts, are afflicted by liberal biases.

It is true that a majority of scientists who work in universities in the United States tend to self-identify as liberal or as Democrats.[5] But the leap from this fact to the conclusion that "we can't trust the scientists" is unwarranted for two reasons. First, political bias, whether on the Left or the Right, is more likely to be present, or to be dispositive, only in certain areas of inquiry, namely, those that have a more direct bearing on the political issues that divide the Left and Right. For example, one should be considerably more vigilant regarding evidence of bias in social science work on the effectiveness or ineffectiveness of welfare programs than work in quantum physics. Second, and more important, the charge that science has a liberal bias completely overlooks the fact that a large part of what distinguishes science from other ways of forming beliefs is that it includes norms and practices *explicitly designed to reduce the risk of bias.* These run the gamut from measures for avoiding use of biased data samples, to double-blind experiments, to the requirement of replicability of results, to the competition for funding and prestige, which gives scientists powerful incentives to expose bias in the work of other scientists.[6]

The point about the bias-correcting function of competition for prestige and funding warrants elaboration. Critics of science find the fact that scientists are often motivated by self-interest to be a disturbing revelation (and a profound insight on their part). One would only have this reaction if one naïvely believed that scientists are not like the rest of humanity (note the parallel with the equally ignorant assumption that individuals "in the public sector" are motivated solely by concern for the common good). The point is not that scientists must be pure of heart if science is to be reliable but that, *as an institution, science tends to harness self-interest in productive ways,* in part through encouraging competition for prestige and funding that often takes the form of younger scientists making their reputation by attacking the status quo view.[7]

The proper response to the risk of bias is not to abandon science but to strengthen its already impressive measures for reducing that risk and embedding them in the relevant institutions. In the case at hand, this would

5. Mitchell Langbert, "Homogenous: The Political Affiliations of Elite Liberal Arts College Faculty," *Academic Questions* 31 (2018): 186–97.

6. Philip Kitcher, "The Cognitive Division of Labor," *The Journal of Philosophy* 87, no. 1 (1990): 5–22.

7. Here I recall Robert O. Keohane's remark that part of what motivates him to be careful about what he publishes is the thought that "there's a dissertation out there with my name on it." Bob also says that what's important is not to have been right, but to be right. (Personal conversations, 2006.)

mean chiefly three things: (1) creating mechanisms that empower dissenting scientific voices *during* the policy-formation process, (2) mandating periodic critical reviews of institutional behavior, with participation by credentialed experts, including an in-depth critical review *after* a crisis has passed, and (3) ensuring that officials provide plausible public justifications of their policies, with a legal duty to respond to critics. In Chapter Four, I develop these recommendations for institutional reform in considerable detail.

There is one more point to be made about bias in science and in the university as a whole. Many scientists and scholars actually have a professional ethic that *does* influence their behavior to some extent. This ethic includes a commitment to the truth and that in turn entails a commitment to self-criticism, even to deliberately seeking out the most serious challenges to one's own beliefs. I can give you an example from my own early career.

When I was a first-year graduate student, John Rawls's *A Theory of Justice* burst upon the academic scene, getting immediate attention not just in philosophy but in political science, sociology, and economics, too. Without too much exaggeration I can say it was like the dramatic scene in *2001: A Space Odyssey*, in which the sudden arrival of a monolith from an advanced civilization prompts a leap in the cognitive development of some rather dim prehuman primates. Similarly, upon reading Rawls's book, the rather intellectually primitive, not overly luminous, unprestigous community of political philosophers suddenly concluded that the history of their discipline wasn't over and began to think independently rather than just digging up skeletons in the graveyard of the history of ideas.

I was overwhelmed by Rawls's views. It all seemed largely right. But that really worried me. I feared that Rawls's principles seemed valid to me because they conveniently fit my biases. So I asked myself: where would I find the deepest challenge to Rawls's kind of philosophy? The answer was obvious: Karl Marx.

So I tuned up my German, ploughed through most of the fifty or so volumes of Marx's collected works, read a lot of secondary literature, and tried to figure out what the best Marxian criticisms of a liberal position like Rawls's were. The result was my first book, *Marx and Justice: The Radical Critique of Liberalism*.[8] I didn't become a Marxist and I didn't reject everything in Rawls. But I think I did achieve a more balanced view. This kind of voluntary self-criticism occurs frequently. Intellectual integrity requires it.

---

8. Allen Buchanan, *Marx and Justice: The Radical Critique of Liberalism* (Totowa, NJ: Roman and Littlefield, 1982).

Some criticisms of the claims of scientific knowledge made by public health authorities during the pandemic are based on another mistaken belief, in addition to the simplistic belief that because scientists are liberal they are biased: that genuine science is "value free" but that the public health enterprise is not. This complaint is based on a naïvely crude understanding of science. Science is not value-free in at least two respects. First, values—more specifically, the beliefs of researchers and of those who fund them about what is important—inevitably shape the choice of items to include in research agendas. Scientists don't (and couldn't) investigate all phenomena: a value filter determines which ones are prioritized. Not all research projects are fundable; only those that funders think important will receive support. And what a scientist or a funder regards as important enough to be the object of scientific study is not determined by science; it is determined by values that people bring to science.

There is a second, deeper sense in which science is not value-free. As I noted in Chapter One, there is a basic epistemic norm, a norm regarding the search for evidence and the formation of hypotheses on the basis of evidence, that plays an important role in scientific reasoning and that explicitly relies on values. This is the principle according to which the greater the risk of accepting a hypothesis, the more robust the evidence in favor of accepting it should be. The point is that what counts as a significant risk and how serious a risk is depends upon what is valuable—more specifically, on what goods will be imperiled if one acts on an hypothesis that turns out to be false. In other words, it is a mistake to think that science only includes epistemic values, not moral values; or rather, the distinction between epistemic norms and moral norms is blurry. Yet it is important to emphasize that although science is not "value-free" for these two reasons (values motivate the choice of objects of scientific study and what counts as sufficient evidence for an hypothesis depends on values) this does not mean that science is "just a matter of subjective preferences" and therefore is not our best available engine for the creation of knowledge.

The bottom line is that if they are to be credible, scientists (including public health experts) must learn to communicate uncertainty and the fallibility of scientific reasoning, as well as the fact that science is not "value free" and is subject to biases. And they must do so in such a manner as to enhance, rather than undermine, their credibility. There are two extremes to be avoided: pretending certainty when humility is appropriate and being so humble as to suggest that science is just a matter of opinion. In my judgment, public health messaging during the COVID-19 pandemic has frequently failed by erring in the direction of lack of humility.

WHY POLICY STATEMENTS AREN'T MATTERS OF SCIENTIFIC EXPERTISE: THE INESCAPABILILTY OF TRADE-OFFS AND, HENCE, OF JUDGMENTS OF COMPARATIVE VALUE

So far, I have emphasized that science is not value-free, is fallible, and usually does not speak with one voice. Now I want to show that policy choices, so far as they are at all supported by reasons, are not matters of purely scientific judgment, but inevitably include controversial moral judgments that do not fall within the expertise of scientists, including public health authorities. The reason that policy choices include an irreducible moral component is that, so far as these choices are reasoned, they embody trade-offs among conflicting values that can only be determined by recourse to moral values or principles.

Here are two examples to show that policy choices are not just scientific matters, but include controversial moral assumptions about how trade-offs are to be made when values conflict.

1. Lockdowns of non-essential businesses, combined with school closings and travel bans, are necessary if we are to slow the spread of the virus. Therefore, we are recommending these measures.
2. The best strategy for coping with COVID-19 include multiple vaccinations plus two or more boosters for as much of the population as possible. Therefore, we must vaccinate and boost as many Americans as possible.

The first example assumes not only that the proposed measures will slow the spread of the virus (a scientific prediction) but also that slowing the spread of the virus is an overriding priority—with the implicit assumption that the delay in the spread of the virus that these measures will achieve is so important that it is worth whatever costs those measures will entail. But to say that slowing the spread of the virus through these measures is worth whatever costs this involves is to make a comparative judgment with an irreducible moral element: to assert that the gain from slowing the spread of the virus is more important than the costs (especially the costs in terms of human welfare and freedom) of doing so.

Clearly, slowing the spread of the virus is not in itself of any value; it is only instrumentally valuable insofar as it will avoid overload of the medical system or have some other good effects. But this means that in recommending measures to slow the spread of the virus, public health authorities are assuming—merely assuming, not demonstrating—that avoiding the damage to the medical system that will be achieved by these measures is more important than avoiding the economic and psychosocial damage the measures will do. That is a moral judgment and a very controversial one. It is a trade-off judgment: an implicit claim that the benefits of the policy exceed its costs. It is an implicit comparative evaluation, not a scientific judgment, as all trade-off judgments are. It endorses "trading" a great deal of economic and psychosocial damage for slowing the spread of the virus and assumes this "trade" is a good bargain. And whether or not it is a good bargain depends upon what is most important, not upon the scientifically ascertainable facts.

By focusing its public communications only on the supposed benefits of school closings, business lockdowns, and travel bans, public health authorities and presidential spokespersons failed to acknowledge that they were making trade-off judgments—judgments that require controversial moral assumption, judgments for which they had no expertise. Instead, they pretended that they were only relying on the scientific prediction that these measures would slow the spread of the virus while encouraging the mistaken idea that all that mattered was to slow the spread so as to avoid strain on the medical system.

To put the same point differently, they proceeded as if there was a trade-off only in a very peculiar sense: no amount of damage from the measures proposed was important enough to justify settling for anything less than the *maximal* possible delay in the spread of the virus. That is, the public health authorities proceeded as if the value of slowing the spread of the virus was so overwhelming that no consideration of costs should constrain the pursuit of this goal in any way. This was irrational. A more reasonable option would be to balance the value of slowing the spread of the virus against the costs of doing so and settle for something less than maximal delay in the spread of the virus. In effect, policymakers accorded unlimited value to slowing the spread of the virus and no disvalue to the harmful effects of pursuing maximal delay. And they did so under the pretense that the policy they recommended was mandated by "the science."

Example 2 above assumes, without good reason, that vaccinating and boosting virtually the whole population is the right policy goal. In doing so it fails to ask a pertinent question: would a vaccination and booster goal somewhat less ambitious be better, all things considered? This question is important to ask because the ambitious goal is costly and the question arises as to whether the benefits of pursuing it are worth the costs.

It is true that the marginal cost of producing a vaccine dose is negligible, but that is only the least important cost factor. Vaccinating and boosting virtually the whole population is very costly: there are the costs of storing and distributing doses, the cost of providing trained medical personnel to administer the doses, and the costs of taking time off from work and other valued activities to get vaccinated and boosted. Given these costs, one needs to consider whether a somewhat less ambitious goal might be better. Once again, what the public got was only one side of a cost-benefit analysis: a claim about the supposed benefits of a policy, with no mention of costs. Without an accounting of costs, one cannot even begin to make a reasonable trade-off judgment. However, in example 2, while the "justification" for a massive vaccination effort implicitly embodies a trade-off, it is an extreme one: the benefits of the proposed policy are assumed to be so great that the costs don't matter. That is a trade-off in which one value is given infinite weight and the opposing value is given zero weight—a very degenerate case of a trade-off judgment. Had it been made explicit, its absurdity would have been apparent.

Here an analogy may prove useful. Suppose the goal is to make automobiles safer. If one focused only on achieving the *maximal* improvement in safety, without regard to costs, one might propose that automobiles be equipped with thick armor and that their engines be down-regulated so that they could only travel at ten miles an hour. If such vehicles were the rule, deaths and serious injuries from car crashes might be around zero. But the costs of these measures would be prohibitive: cars would be so expensive (due to the cost of armor plating) and so slow that much of the value of having a car would be lost. Safety is a concern, but the trade-off between safety, on the one hand, an affordability and convenience, on the other, should accord considerable value to both sides of the equation rather than treating safety as an absolute, indeed infinite value.

Economics provides another way to frame the essential point: the marginal costs of risk reduction tend to rise and that must be taken into account in making rational trade-off judgments. Consider again the car example: for every added inch of armor plating, one gets a corresponding increment of risk reduction. But at a certain point the cheap risk reduction has already occurred and each additional increment of reduction is more costly and eventually too costly, with the increments of risk-reduction dwindling, given that we value other things than safety. To assume that all that matters is maximizing risk reduction is to ignore this crucial point.

When designing policy, acknowledging that the marginal costs of risk reduction tend to increase is only one aspect, though an important one, of a rational approach to trade-offs. I find it remarkable that if one did not have the concept of trade-offs or of the increasing marginal costs of risk reduction, nothing in the public communications of the CDC would have made you aware of these basic ideas. They simply were not part of the vocabulary employed by public health authorities in their announcements of policies. That is because that discourse focused only on the supposed benefits of policies, with no consideration of costs. And this egregious omission meant that there was nothing approaching a sound public justification for pandemic policies.

Having the right policies is important, but not enough: one also needs to justify them to the public. This is a *moral* requirement as well as a *prudential* one: moral because citizens in a democracy ought to be treated as beings to whom reasons matter; prudential because the absence of justification encourages poor decision-making that eventually undermines the authority of those who fail to provide reasonable justifications. Further, bearing the burden of a public justification is important for ascertaining whether the policy one is proposing really is the right policy. A plausible justification counts in favor of the policy, the inability to produce a plausible justification is an indicator that the policy is not a good one. Conscientious policymakers will submit themselves to the discipline of providing a public justification for the policies they propose.

JUSTIFICATION AND RESPECT
FOR PERSONS AS REASONABLE BEINGS

There is a deeper reason why policymakers owe the public reasonable justifications for policies that affect their welfare and freedom, a reason that is not limited to the requirements of respecting the public as citizens in a democracy, in which officials are supposed to be accountable to the public: it is required if officials are to acknowledge the fundamental equal basic moral status of all individuals. An important element of that status is the ability to participate in what philosopher Stephen Darwall calls "the second-person standpoint."[9] We occupy this standpoint when we regard

9. Stephen Darwall, *The Second-Person Standpoint: Morality, Respect, and Accountability* (Cambridge, MA: Harvard University Press, 2006).

ourselves and others as "reasonable" beings, as creatures that are responsive to reasons and who acknowledge that so far as our behavior affects others we bear a burden of justification. In brief, showing respect for persons requires adopting this second person or "we" perspective, the recognition that we are engaged in an enterprise that demonstrates mutual respect through responsiveness to reasons. The profound German philosopher Rainer Forst develops this idea more systematically: all persons, he says, as persons, have a fundamental "right to justification."[10]

In the case of policymakers, basic respect for those who will be subject to their policies requires a sincere effort to provide a plausible public justification for those policies. To fail to do so is to treat the public as less than persons, as less than reasonable beings, in effect denying that one owes them reasons for what one is requiring of them. To issue policy directives without public justifications is to treat people as if they were not reasonable beings, but rather are objects to be managed or children who are to obey. I develop this point in Chapter Four.

Some economists have suggested that they, not public health officials, are the experts on determining the trade-offs that pandemic policy choices inevitably require. It is true that economists recognize the need to make trade-offs, and that is to their credit. And they are correct to point out that public health expertise is not sufficient to ground policy judgments, so far as these involve trade-offs that can only be determined by a comparison of values. But they are wrong if they go farther and hold that trade-offs are to be determined solely by economic expertise and, more specifically, by the economist's expertise regarding efficiency.

Fortunately, most economists now recognize that their expertise is necessary but not sufficient for making reasonable trade-offs. Once a policy goal is specified, they can use their skills as economists to tell us how to achieve it most efficiently. But economic reasoning alone cannot specify the goal; and specifying the goal typically requires making trade-off judgments.

Modern economics operates with several related conceptions of efficiency. The most widely employed is Pareto Optimality: a state of a given system is Pareto Optimal if and only if there is no alternative feasible state of that system in which at least one individual is better off and no one is worse off. A state S1 is Pareto Superior to another state S2 if and only if at

10. Rainer Forst, *The Right to Justification: Elements of a Constructivist Theory of Justice*, translated by Jeffrey Flynn (New York: Columbia University Press, 2014).

least one individual is better off in S₁ than in S₂ and no one is worse off in S₁ than in S₂. The Pareto Optimality and Pareto Superiority principles appear to provide the most comprehensive tools for assessing efficiency, because the notion of a social state they employ is inclusive enough to take into account the way productive resources are allocated, the way production is organized, and the distribution of goods so far as this affects how well off individuals are.

The wide acceptance of the Pareto Optimality and Pareto Superiority principles among economists is due at least in part to the fact that they provide a way of assessing social states that does not require defensible interpersonal utility comparisons. Interpersonal utility comparisons require a common scale on which the utilities of all affected individuals can be located, so that an overall net score, aggregating utilities and disutilities can be calculated. "Utility" here is understood to be the satisfaction of preferences, with the additional (and highly questionable) assumption that well-being is a matter of the satisfaction of preferences.

Perhaps the predominant account of why interpersonal utility comparisons cannot be made is that they require something that cannot be provided, namely, a nonarbitrary way of selecting a common zero point for the single scale on which all individual's utilities are to be located. For many economists, the attraction of the Pareto Optimality and Pareto Superiority principles is that they are a second-best alternative to what would be optimal if available, namely, utility maximization.

In addition to the fact that most controversial policies produce losers as well as winners and that consequently there is no Pareto Optimal option, the Paretian efficiency principles are subject to a fundamental limitation: a state of affairs can be efficient, yet grossly unfair or inequitable. To take an extreme example: a state of affairs in which a small minority enslaves the majority could be Pareto efficient—it might be impossible to improve the lot of the slaves without worsening the condition of the slaveholders. The general point is that Paretian efficiency is distributionally insensitive. And because whether distributions are fair or equitable matters, Paretian efficiency is not a sufficient tool for evaluating policies.

In brief, although efficiency matters, it is not all that matters, because an efficient state of affairs can be morally unacceptable. Further, sometimes a trade-off between efficiency and equity is in order. But if that is so, then we have a second reason why appealing to efficiency cannot provide a sufficient way to determine all trade-offs.

Some economists—happily, a dwindling minority—still wrongly assume that (Pareto) efficiency is *the* appropriate way to determine trade-offs, that efficient trade-offs are the only rational ones. In making this assumption, they are either failing to notice that other values, including fairness or equity, are relevant to determining trade-offs; or they are implicitly assuming the truth of a highly controversial moral theory, namely, utilitarianism, according to which the overriding moral principle is to maximize overall utility, and treating Paretian efficiency as a second best for utility maximization. The latter error is apparent in the following quotation from the eminent public choice economist, Gordon Tullock, in his book *The Logic of the Law*: "In this book I will eschew moral arguments, appealing only to utility."[11] Consider now a second quote, this time from an article by Peter Boettke and Benjamin Powell advocating an economic approach to COVID-19 policy: "Economics is the science that deals with evaluating the trade-offs between costs and benefits."[12]

Tullock's quote indicates a stunning failure to recognize that to hold that all that matters is utility maximization is to assume the validity of the moral theory known as utilitarianism, while failing to recognize that it *is* a moral theory and a much disputed one at that. Perhaps the strongest evidence that one has *uncritically* adopted a moral theory—in this case utilitarianism—is that one is completely unaware that one has adopted it or takes its truth to be self-evident.

The second quote, from Boettke and Powell, strongly suggests that considerations of efficiency are sufficient for making trade-off judgments and therefore that, since economists are experts on efficiency, economic expertise is sufficient for making trade-off judgments. At one point the authors of the second quote do acknowledge that "equity" (a term they find so problematic that they frame it in scare quotes) may matter, but that it can be taken into account by redistributing income after the efficient way of allocating costs and benefits has been achieved.

Any microeconomist worthy of the title knows that using markets and the price system is usually the best way to allocate scarce resources to maximize value. If some "equity" goal, or wealth constraint, is the concern, economists have long recognized that it is more efficient to

11. Gordon Tullock, *The Logic of the Law* (New York: Basic Books, 1971), chap. 1.

12. Peter Boettke and Benjamin Powell, "The Political Economy of the COVID-19 Pandemic," *Southern Economic Journal* 87, no. 4 (2021): 1090–1106.

redistribute resources through income transfers, than to make direct allocations, in-kind, of a scarce good.[13]

Although the quote refers to the allocation of scarce goods, the point about ex-post redistribution is a more general one, the idea being that equity concerns, or other moral constraints on the pursuit of efficiency, can be handled by ex-post redistribution.

Relying on ex-post redistribution to handle equity concerns is problematic for two reasons. First, not all costs (e.g., death) can be fully compensated for with ex-post cash transfers). Second, and more importantly, the ex-post redistribution strategy assumes a falsehood, namely that how things get produced and initially distributed in a society does not constrain the feasible options for ex-post redistribution. The point is that the ways in which goods are produced and initially distributed express, perpetuate, and in some cases increase power disparities, with the result that the better off predictably block attempts to rectify inequities after the fact through policies that require them to transfer some of their wealth to the less powerful. In brief, in the real world, distribution is not independent of production.

Responding to the fact that efficient policies can be inequitable or otherwise morally defective by saying that these defects can be remedied ex post through redistribution is a remarkably idealistic pronouncement by supposedly realistic economists. In effect, it assumes that the prospects for redistribution will not be shaped by the self-interest of the better off but instead will be determined by a sincere commitment to equity.

Put differently, it assumes that the state (the agent of redistribution) is exogenous to the economy and that state agents, including legislators, can be counted on to violate the fundamental principle of public choice theory, according to which actors in the public sector are not radically different from people elsewhere. The quote endorsing the ex-post redistribution strategy is especially ironic, considering that it appears in an article whose title is "The Political Economy of the COVID-19 Pandemic," and which states that political economy "starts from a basic behavioral postulate that people are the same whether they are in the marketplace, the government or the non-profit voluntary sector."[14] The ex-post redistributive strategy assumes that the principles of political economy apply

13. Boettke and Powell, "The Political Economy of the COVID-19 Pandemic," 1098.
14. Boettke and Powell, "The Political Economy of the COVID-19 Pandemic."

everywhere *except* to the politics of redistribution. The economists' answer to the objection that efficiency is not all that matters and that efficient outcomes can be morally defective comes at the price of a gross inconsistency in their assumptions about human motivation.

If one abandons the hyperidealistic psychological assumptions of the ex-post redistribution strategy, the only alternative appears to be to try to take equity (distributional fairness) and other relevant moral values into account in determining policy, rather than ignoring their relevance until it is too late and relying on ex-post redistribution. But if that is so, then it is not true that economic expertise is sufficient for determining trade-offs. The hard work of making the needed moral judgments remains; and economic expertise is not sufficient for doing it. Economists, qua economists, can only tell us how to achieve our goals once they have been specified, and specifying them requires making trade-offs that cannot be determined solely by considerations of efficiency or any other economic criterion. That means that economists, like public health experts, have special skills that are necessary but not sufficient for making reasonable trade-offs.

Given my conclusions thus far, (1) that policies, if they are supportable by reasons, always at least implicitly assume trade-offs, and (2) that determining trade-offs requires not just efficiency assessments or scientific judgments but also moral reasoning, the question arises: Who has the relevant expertise? At the risk of sounding self-serving, I suggest that moral philosophers have a contribution to make. They are "moral experts" only in the sense that they routinely articulate the premises of moral arguments, distinguish different moral values, and grapple with the problem of how to resolve conflicts among values. My suggestion is that the optimal arrangement would be to include both economists and moral philosophers accustomed to work in "practical ethics," along with public health experts, of course, in an interdisciplinary approach to formulating policies for preparing for the next pandemic. But whether I am right to think that moral philosophers have something to contribute, I think I have conclusively established that policy formation, so far as it includes trade-offs, does not fall within the expertise either of public health experts or economists.

Here it might be objected that there is no need for moral expertise: policy goals and the trade-off judgments they reflect should be determined by democratic political processes. No doubt that is true, but the fact remains that serious efforts should be made to ensure that those processes are guided, not just by proper public health and economic expertise, or by unreflective majority opinion, but by sound moral reasoning. The question is whether we can develop ways of ensuring that this happens. There have been changes in this direction regarding morally fraught policy in other areas, most notably the creation of a new institution, the presidential bio-ethics commission. In the current pandemic, although both presidential administrations have consulted with interdisciplinary groups, there has been no clear recognition that there are distinct types of expertise that are relevant for determining pandemic policy and that each has its limitations.

I conclude this chapter by emphasizing that the misrepresentation of expertise that has characterized U.S. official responses to the COVID-19 pandemic is not just a theoretical error. It has serious negative practical consequences. Most importantly, it provides officials with a means of deflecting valid criticisms, by enabling them to claim that those who challenge their policies lack the qualifications to do so. In addition, by disguising controversial moral assumptions as judgments of technical expertise, it obscures the nature of the reasoning that led to specific policy choices and undercuts the prospects for providing reasonable justifications for them. Finally, by failing to acknowledge the limits of their expertise, public health officials wrongly extend their power over us and deprive us of our proper role in determining how to respond to a pandemic or other health crisis. The same loss of agency on the part of the public would occur if economists successfully misrepresented the extent of their expertise. Power based on fraudulent claims of expertise is usurpation. It unjustly enhances the power of the experts while at the same time disempowering all of us.[15]

---

15. The CDC did acknowledge the relevance of moral values in the case of decisions regarding the allocation of vaccine doses, stating that allocation should be guided, inter alia, by the effort to "maximize benefits and minimize harms.... mitigate health injustices.... promote justice.... promote transparency." See https://www.cdc.gov/coronavirus/2019-ncov /vaccines/recommendations-process.html. No effort was made, however, to explain to the public how particular policies exemplified these principles; nor was there any acknowledgment that they could be in conflict, necessitating trade-offs. In brief, this was a ritualistic invocation of a list of abstract values, with no effort to demonstrate how they were being put to work in policy decisions. Further, it is clearly not enough to assert that benefits should be maximized and harms minimized. What is needed is an explicit cost-benefit analysis, with the results and evidential bases made publicly available.

THREE

Pandemic Politics

I noted in Chapter One that the politics of the pandemic occur in three distinct domains: (1) the internal politics of the highest-level public health agencies, in the U.S. case the CDC, FDA, and HHS; (2) the impact on these agencies of organized political forces coming from outside them; and (3) the larger, society-wide political environment in which the pandemic is occurring, an environment I characterize as tribalistic. My focus in this chapter is mainly on the third domain. I have already provided, in Chapter Two, the bare bones of an account of the first and second domains. More specifically, I have noted that the CDC, HHS, and FDA, like other large-scale, hierarchical organizations, are subject to political behavior in their internal workings, and that consequntly the public ought to take seriously the possibility that internal politics may hinder the organization's performance. And I have noted that the Executive Branch has exerted undue influence on policymakers.

INTRAORGANIZATIONAL POLITICS

Recall that a standard definition of politics is the struggle for power. Organizations are sites of the struggle for power. Those at the top of the organizational hierarchy generally seek to preserve and enhance their power, and those below them generally want to increase their power in the positions they currently hold while gaining more power through rising higher in the organizational hierarchy. In both cases, success depends on making bargains, accumulating debts, calling them in, and forging coalitions. Even those individuals who do not seek power must act strategically, defensively taking into account the maneuvers of those who do, if they are to avoid demotion or limitations on their ability to do what they think they should do.

This is not to say that most people seek power for its own sake, as an ultimate end. Instead, they typically regard power as instrumentally valuable for the achievement of whatever ends they have. And in the case of public organizations, the ends, in many cases, may be different from the ends of individuals in private organizations. They may include the public welfare, which may be accorded considerable priority.[1]

As I noted in Chapter One, organizations like the CDC are both highly prestigious and monopolistic. They feature especially strong incentives for conformity, for subordinates not challenging their superiors. Because the leaders of the organization are not elected and are not subject to term limits, they can accumulate a great deal of power over time—power not constrained by accountability to those lower in the hierarchy. This set of conditions is a recipe for excessive loyalty and uncritical conformity because challenging those at the top of the hierarchy is likely to be not only costly but also ineffective. Such organizations therefore may be especially prone to the "yes men" phenomenon that is a risk in all hierarchical organizations—unless there are specific mechanisms designed to empower dissenting views. The key point is that the workings of the internal politics of the top-level public health agencies are not automatically aligned with the effective pursuit of the organization's mission; they can in fact detract from it.

Our understanding of the internal politics of major public health institutions is enhanced if we utilize a fruitful and justly famous distinction drawn by Albert O. Hirschman.[2] Hirschman identifies three archetypal

---

1. I have not had recourse to public choice theory in my characterization of pandemic politics because I think that it exaggerates an important point. While it is true that one should not attribute extreme altruism or vastly superior knowledge to people in the public sector, it is equally mistaken to assume that, on average, there are no differences in the motivation between a person working in a profit-maximizing firm and another who could have occupied that sort of position but chose instead to work for a human rights organization and much greater personal risk and with greatly inferior financial compensation. While it is true that individuals, or at least most of them, in both public and private organizations seek power as something of great instrumental value, the ends they use it to pursue can be quite different. My analysis allows for significant motivational differences regarding public versus private agents, but it still takes seriously the fact that public institutional performance is subject to adverse political influences that also exist in the private sphere. One need not assume the truth of public choice theory to make the case that there was serious institutional failure in the current pandemic.

2. Albert O. Hirschman, *Exit, Voice, and Loyalty* (Cambridge, MA: Harvard University Press, 1972).

responses that members of an organization can utilize when they find themselves at odds with organizational policy: exit, loyalty, and voice. The highest, national-level public health agencies are monopolies; hence there is no possibility of exit to a rival institution of the same importance and power. For those who have chosen a career in public health, being employed at the national level may well be the ultimate goal. For such persons, exit may not be a serious option.

By the loyalty option, Hirschman means swallowing one's disagreement and continuing to cooperate as usual. There are certainly strong incentives for members of top public health agencies to take this route; doing so ensures continuation of employment and the exceptionally generous benefits that go with their position. In addition, agreeing with rather than challenging one's superiors is more likely to gain their support for being promoted.

The attraction of the loyalty option is enhanced if one considers that the voice option may be both very costly to exercise (one may be regarded as disloyal, as not a team player) *and* unlikely to affect the behavior of the powerful, unelected top officials toward whom it would be directed, due to the fact that there are no effective mechanisms for holding them accountable, for ensuring that dissenting voices actually affect their behavior. Because the leaders of the CDC and HHS have accumulated power over decades, the most adaptive behavior for those below them in the hierarchy will often be not to question their judgment and, what is worse, to say what their superiors want to hear. The proper response to this "yes man" phenomenon is not to tell those lower down in the hierarchy to pull up their moral socks and sacrifice their careers; it is to adopt specific institutional measures to empower them and reduce the costs of their exercising the voice option.

EXTERNAL POLITICAL INFLUENCE

One of the most important features of the second domain of politics is the fact that the heads of the top-level public health agencies in the United States are formally answerable to Congress, upon whom they depend for funding. Although I do not pretend to have hard data to back this hypothesis up, my conjecture is that, during the present pandemic, Congress was largely supportive of the policies of the CDC and HHS or at least did not make serious efforts to change or thwart them. This would not be surprising if Congress, like much of the public, accepted the public health expert's inflated claims of expertise. Whether Congress will conduct serious, well-designed hearings to make a critical appraisal of these agencies' behavior in the pandemic at some later date, after the pandemic is regarded as over, remains to be seen. If anything, Congress was too passive, to accepting of problematic public health policies.

As noted earlier, there were two egregious instances of presidential meddling in COVID-19 policy. In the first, President Donald J. Trump succeeded temporarily in influencing FDA policy without having the authority to do so. He pressured the HHS to urge the FDA Commissioner to accord Emergency Use Authorization (EUA) status for Hydroxychloroquine, a drug that later extensive studies proved to be inefficacious in the treatment of COVID-19 and unsafe as well.[3] The FDA Commissioner wrongly caved in to this inappropriate intervention, but later backtracked, revoking the EUA. In the second instance, as I noted in Chapter One, the Biden administration pressured the FDA to approve the use of anti-COVID-19 vaccines in very young children, in spite of the fact that efficacy was low or nonexistent and that there was a risk of serious negative effects on children's long-term health and development that could not be ascertained by the studies undertaken. It is worth noting that some other countries, including Sweden, have legal barriers between political officials and public health institutions, forbidding the former to intervene in decisions made in the latter. The United States lacks such measures.

It might be thought that the prospect of congressional disapproval would create a significant degree of accountability and exert an influence in the direction of sound policy. Whether that is the case depends, however, on three factors: (1) whether members of Congress believe themselves qualified to challenge the judgment of public health officials at the highest level, (2) whether Congress has access to independent sources of information about the performance of the agencies in question, and (3) whether members of Congress are concerned primarily with helping to ensure sound policies or have other priorities, such as being reelected or enhancing their power in Congress. All three of these assumptions are problematic.

To the extent that public health officials succeed in promulgating the myth that policy decisions are wholly within the scope of their expertise and control the information about what they are doing that is available to Congress, this potentially important mode of accountability may be of

---

3. See Scott Gottlieb, *Uncontrolled Spread: Why COVID-19 Crushed Us and How We Can Defeat the Next Pandemic* (New York: Harper Collins, 2021), 292–96.

little consequence. The information problem here is a general one: institutional insiders have greater knowledge of what they are doing than outsiders do. Unless there is a great deal of transparency as to the actual operations of the institution, along with mechanisms for transmitting relevant information in understandable terms to outsiders, this asymmetry of knowledge will seriously limit accountability. When the lack of effective measures to overcome the insider/outsider information asymmetry is combined with inappropriate deference to supposed insider expertise, merely formal accountability will be inadequate.

THE TRIBALISTIC POLITICIZATION OF THE PANDEMIC

Much more troubling is the third domain of politics, the ways in which the toxic environment of political tribalism that characterizes the United States today distorts public and private responses to the pandemic. Here I advance three theses. First, because tribalism is totalizing, transforming every area of social life into a contest between Us and Them, behavior that should have been evaluated on the merits becomes an emblem of allegiance to one tribe and rejection of another. Second, the tribalistic mentality corrupts public discourse, making rational deliberation impossible, chiefly by shifting attention from an evaluation of the content of what is said to an evaluation of the speaker's tribal affiliation. Third, tribalism contributes to erosion of the institutional legitimacy that is necessary for an effective response to the next pandemic. It undermines legitimacy by replacing attempts to make reasonable assessments of institutional performance with sorting and signaling—sorting actors into Us versus Them and using discourse to signal allegiance to our group—rather than to contribute to a genuine exchange of relevant reasons. To support these claims, it is first necessary to provide a clear and detailed exposition of what I mean by "tribalism," distinguishing it both from the more general (and often benign) human tendency to "groupishness" and from "political polarization."[4]

Humans are groupish animals. We tend to divide the social world along in-group and out-group lines and show marked partiality toward our own group. Further, for most people, group membership is an important type or element of identity. It may be that this tendency to groupishness is the basis of tribalism, but tribalism, as I make clear below, is groupishness

---

4. Allen Buchanan, *Our Moral Fate: Evolution and the Escape from Tribalism* (Cambridge, MA: MIT Press, 2020).

in an extreme and profoundly destructive form, one in which outgroup members are dehumanized and regarded as implacable enemies.

Polarization is usefully defined as the presence of deep and increasing disagreements on important social and political issues. The key point is that polarization, unlike tribalism, is compatible with respect for those one disagrees with, and with a commitment to compromise and bargaining.

So what do I mean by tribalism? Tribalism is a style of thinking, a set of attitudes, and a practical orientation to the social world that includes the following features.

1. All important social and political issues are bundled together in what is conceived as a no-holds-barred, zero-sum struggle for the highest stakes, a Supreme Emergency that is a life-or-death struggle between good and evil. Consequently, tribalism is totalizing: everything, from what kind of car one drives to whether one wears a mask in a pandemic, becomes a partisan issue. More accurately, all issues and all behaviors are political, insofar as we define the political as the struggle for power—in the case of tribalism, the struggle for power between Us and Them.

2. The division between Us and Them is exhaustive: if you are not one of Us, you are one of Them, the implacable enemy of all that is good and right. Any disagreement with the beliefs that define Us puts one ask risk of being regarded as one of Them.

3. There is no common ground between Us and Them, no room for meeting in the middle, for bargaining and compromise, because it is a matter of absolute good versus absolute evil. This belief undermines democracy, because for democracy to work citizens must regard each other as potential parties to compromise, as beings with whom on can bargain. Above all, democracy only works if citizens are confident that if they lose today on an issue, they may win tomorrow. This crucial tenet of democratic faith is extinguished by the tribalistic view that all political issues are bound together in a winner takes all, zero-sum, life-or-death struggle.

4. The Other—all of Them—are either irremediably misinformed and stupid or irredeemably insincere and untrustworthy. Hence one cannot reason with them; nothing they say is either worth attending to or to be taken at face value. This means that rational engagement with the Other is impossible. So far as we include the idea of

rationality, of being able to reason, in our conception of humanity, the Other is therefore less than human.

5. Because rational discourse between Us and Them is impossible, given that the Other is not a being capable of reasoning, discourse degenerates into "sorting and signaling": sorting people into Us versus Them and signaling one's membership in and unalloyed allegiance to one's group. What appear to be reports of states of belief (e.g., "If Biden is elected, he will make this a communist country") do convey information, but not about what one actually believes will happen; instead, the information conveyed is the signal that one is not a Democrat but rather is a Republican and a Trump supporter. However, what begins as a mere signal of allegiance can become a belief.

6. The tribalistic posture on the beliefs held by Our group is one of comprehensive certainty: We know the truth on all important issues, and They have nothing to offer, even by way of qualifying those truths. This is another reason why rational engagement with the Other is futile: we have nothing to learn from them. Nor are there any circumstances in which we would be led to revise our views: we now possess the final truth on all matters of importance.

This is a characterization of tribalism as an ideal type, the extreme on a spectrum of beliefs and attitudes that are tribalistic to a greater or lesser degree. My conjecture—and it is little more than that—is that more extreme forms of tribalism drive less extreme forms to extinction in a kind of race to the bottom.

Taken together, these elements of tribalism undermine a fundamental principle that guides the interactions and communications between individuals who regard each other as equals in the sense of being reason-able beings. I refer here to a principle of charitable interpretation: we are to proceed on the assumption that the other person is sincere in what he or she says. Of course, this assumption is defeasible; an individual may demonstrate that she is insincere, that her communications are not trustworthy. But it is quite another thing to proceed in the tribalistic manner, to start with a presumption of insincerity. Acting on this presumption is a self-fulfilling prophecy: by assuming that no genuine communication with the Other is possible, we make it so.

Here are two concrete examples, one from the Right, the other from the Left, of how individuals in the tribalistic mode proceed on the assumption that the Other is not worth listening to, with the result that there is no rational engagement on the substance of issues.

1. The late Rush Limbaugh repeatedly claimed that Liberals really care nothing about immigrants, that they only advocate "open borders" because they believe that immigrants will vote Democratic. By impugning the motives of those he disagrees with, Limbaugh conveniently sidestepped the arguments in favor of fewer restrictions on immigration. He ignored the message by attacking the character of the messenger.
2. Many people on the left flatly refused to consider the possibility that the COVID-19 virus originated in a laboratory accident in Wuhan, China, not because they had reviewed the evidence, but because President Trump had suggested that this was the case. This, too, is an example of failing to engage on substance, by sorting the messenger into the category of the untrustworthy Other.

The replacement of rational debate by sorting into Us versus Them is an example of an epistemic vice, a bad habit regarding the formation of beliefs, namely, the adoption of a posture of extreme deference to supposed authority (the authentic voices of Us), on the one hand, and total discrediting of the testimony of individuals on the grounds of their supposed membership in the vilified group (Them), on the other.

For much of our history, we ignored or discounted the testimony of women or people of color or the poor—instances of the moral wrong Miranda Fricker famously identifies as "testimonial injustice." Now, if we are in the grip of tribalism, we engage in a new form of testimonial injustice: we disregard the testimony of an individual simply because we have classified her as one of Them.[5]

Epistemic deference is necessary in human life, because none of us can know everything on our own. But epistemic deference can be excessive and misplaced. Tribalism includes two fundamental errors regarding epistemic deference. On the one hand, it fosters absolute, unqualified deference to the testimony of those believed to be the proper spokespersons for our group, regarding them as never to be questioned on peril of being branded disloyal. On the other hand, it automatically discredits entirely the testimony of all persons whom we regard as members of the group that is thought to be our

---

5. Miranda Fricker, *Epistemic Injustice* (New York: Oxford University Press, 2007), chap. 1.

implacable enemy. The combined effect of these two epistemic vices is to prevent any rational engagement on the substance of social and political issues. In the case of pandemic policy issues, this means that instead of genuine deliberation, we get signaling of group identity and loyalty. The point of "communication" becomes limited to signaling absolute deference to those who supposedly speak for Us while utterly rejecting everything that They say.

Cognitive psychology includes a concept, namely, "theory of mind," that illuminates the destructive character of tribalism's orientation toward those regarded as the Other. "Theory of mind" refers to the impressive ability of cognitively normal human beings to infer the mental states of other human beings on the basis of their behavior. Tribalism cripples a person's theory of mind. It does so by filtering our interpretation of the meaning of the Other's behavior through a set of assumptions about what all members of the Other are like.

For example, if I am a person of the Right and see a neighbor wearing a mask, I am likely to infer that he is a Liberal, when in fact the more plausible explanation may be that he is elderly and merely being prudent. Once I have sorted an individual into the opposing group, I am no longer capable of making sound inferences about her intentions and beliefs on the basis of her behavior, because my very perception of her behavior is distorted by my assumption of her group membership. In sorting her into a particular group, I assume that she shares an essence, a nature, with all other members of that group and that this essence or nature determines her beliefs and behaviors. "They are all alike; all Conservatives (or Democrats) are the same."

It is because tribalism is so homogenizing in its view of those considered to be members of the menacing Other that it hinders the proper operation of theory of mind. All of Them are assumed to have the same beliefs and motivations, and inferences about the behavior of particular individuals are made on the basis of that assumption. Putting the same point differently, we can say that the sorting function of tribalism attributes the same, deterministic essence to all those we assign to a particular group. This assumption shapes our perception of their behavior and thereby biases our inferences from behavior to mental states.

To take an earlier example, if I think you are a Liberal and that all that Liberals care about is increasing the number of people who vote Democratic, I may systematically misinterpret your statements and actions regarding immigration. My rigid stereotype of what Liberals are like will prevent me from properly inferring what you believe on the basis of your actions and statements—both of which I will systematically misinterpret.

Further, if I assume that your behavior is insincere and dangerous because I have identified you as one of Them, I will most likely act in ways that you will then interpret as hostile and this will cause you to respond accordingly. In this way, the faulty theory of mind that tribalism produces leads to behavior that seems to confirm it misinterpretations.

Tribalism's undercutting of the operation of theory of mind has dire consequences. Figuring out what the other person wants and values and why they are acting as they do is important for being able to engage productively with them, and to bargain and compromise. And bargaining and compromise are essential for democracy.

HOW TRIBALISM UNDERMINES LEGITIMACY

When people regard an institution as legitimate, this makes a difference as to how they behave in relation to it. To regard it as legitimate is to accord it a certain standing or status. In one influential definition, a legitimate institution is one that exercises rightful authority. If the institution is legitimate, then the presumption is that if there are deficiencies, the first resort is to try to reform it rather than to scrap it. And if it is legitimate, then its agents should be accorded a presumption of respect. Further, there is a presumption that the rules or directives of the institution should be complied with by those to whom they are rightly addressed and a presumption that neither they nor others should interfere with the institutions operations. Of course, all of these presumptions are defeasible. If, for example, the institution persists in engaging in activities that undermine its stated mission, it can lose legitimacy.

Legitimacy is a different and in most cases a less demanding standard than justice, though serious and persistent injustice can deprive an institution of legitimacy. Legitimacy is important because institutions can provide important benefits that cannot be reaped without them. Whatever else they do, institutions coordinate the behavior of large numbers of people in beneficial ways.

Institutions cannot achieve coordination—not without dangerous levels of coercion—unless they are widely regarded as legitimate. This means that there is what I have elsewhere called a meta- or second-level coordination problem: institutions cannot deliver the goods that make them valuable, including coordination, unless there is coordinated support of them, the kind of support that comes from regarding them as legitimate.

For this coordinated support to occur without recourse to dangerous levels of coercion, there must be a consensus among a sufficient number of people that the institution possesses rightful authority. But that means there must be consensus on when the institution is good enough to warrant our support, agreement on criteria for legitimacy.

The problem is that when the tribalistic mentality is pervasive, the needed consensus is not likely to be forthcoming. That consensus requires widely shared beliefs about what the institution is like, what it is doing, and what the motivations of the key institutional agents are. We have seen, however, that tribalism distorts the interpretation of behavior and involves radical distrust of the testimony of others. When tribalism takes hold, institutional behavior is not impartially evaluated; instead, the only question becomes: Are the key institutional agents members of our group or are they the enemy Other?

It appears that many institutions in America today—from the Electoral College to the Supreme Court—are no longer perceived to be legitimate by many people. Perceived legitimacy is always fragile but, under conditions of tribalism, the assessment of institutional legitimacy becomes a strictly partisan affair, with the result that there may not be a sufficient consensus on the legitimacy of important institutions.

Indeed, discourse about legitimacy may be completely off target, focusing exclusively on whether an institution's most influential officials are one of Us or one of Them, with no genuine engagement on what the institution's actual performance is. And whatever assessments of institutional performance do occur are likely to be distorted by the defective theory of mind that tribalism fosters. Trust in institutional agents will not exist across tribal divisions.

The key point is that in discourse about institutional legitimacy, as in discourse more generally, tribalism drives out genuine deliberation and makes reason-based convergence of views difficult if not impossible. Yet without a widespread belief in the legitimacy of the relevant institutions, even the best plans for dealing with the next pandemic may not be effectively implemented. It is not much of an exaggeration to say that the single most important resource for coping with the next pandemic is institutional legitimacy and it appears that this resource is dwindling under the onslaught of tribalism. And as I argued in Chapter Two, by misrepresenting their expertise, projecting certainty rather than humility, and failing to provide anything approaching adequate public justifications for their policies, the leadership of American national public health institutions have worsened the legitimacy crisis.

FOUR

The Need for National Institutional Reform

In this chapter I outline much needed institutional changes at the national level. It is important to emphasize at the outset that we are not talking about a single, overarching institution. In the case of the United States, as in many others, there is a complex set of institutions that are responsible for pandemic policy and there is some indeterminacy as to the boundaries of their respective jurisdictions. The institutional changes I am about to recommend are to be understood as applying to the whole complex, but in the light of a reasonable division of labor among the constituent institutions. Most of the changes will apply, however, to each of the institutions that, taken together, determine pandemic policy. Further, the core suggestions for institutional improvement—in particular the requirements of accountability mechanisms and public justifications—apply not just at the national government level but also to more local institutions, including state and municipal governments in the highly decentralized U.S. political order.

The institutional changes I recommend are directed primarily toward two goals: (1) improving the quality of policy decisions by subjecting policymakers to accountability for decisions and (2) helping to remedy the legitimacy deficit that their behavior during the COVID-19 pandemic has helped to create. I propose, however, a deeper rationale for these institutional changes: they are needed if officials are to treat citizens with the equal respect to which they are morally entitled. That is because the most important institutional innovations I propose include concrete provisions requiring officials to address members of the public as persons, as reasonable beings who are owed plausible justifications for the constraints on their freedom and the impact on their interests that official policies entail.

So far, I have only emphasized the practical importance of institutional legitimacy, where "legitimacy" is understood in the sociological sense. When the term is used in this way it refers to the pervasive belief or perception that an institution has a certain standing, that it exercises rightful authority, with the implication that its operations are not to be interfered with, that its agents are owed a kind of impersonal respect by virtue of their institutional roles, and that there is a presumption that those to whom the institution addresses rules ought to comply with them. The crucial point is that there is a distinction between sociological legitimacy, which is a matter of how people regard the institution, and normative legitimacy, which is a matter of the institution actually having rightful authority.

Both sociological and normative legitimacy are important. If an institution lacks sociological legitimacy, it may be forced to rely on dangerous levels of coercion to achieve adequate compliance with its rules and directives. If an institution lacks normative legitimacy, it exercises power arbitrarily and unjustly.

The eminent international relations scholar Robert O. Keohane and I have developed a general account of institutional legitimacy in the normative sense.[1] What we call the complex understanding of normative institutional legitimacy includes the following elements.

1. The processes by which the institution came to be did not involve serious injustices (the *non-usurpation* or *acceptable origins condition*).
2. There is no serious and persistent discrepancy between the official goals or mission of the institution and its actual behavior (the *institutional integrity condition*).
3. The operations of the institution do not involve serious and persisting violations of basic rights (the *minimal morality condition*).
4. The institution provides significant benefits over and above those that are available without it (the *comparative benefit condition*).
5. The institution has plausible mechanisms for correcting errors over time.

1. Allen Buchanan and Robert O. Keohane, "The Legitimacy of Global Governance Institutions," *Ethics & International Affairs* 20, no. 4 (2006): 405–37.

These conditions are not offered as being individually necessary for normative legitimacy. Rather, the more of them that are satisfied and the greater the extent to which they are satisfied, the more substantial is the institution's claim to exercise rightful authority. The basic concept is that these conditions specify what an institution must be like for it to warrant our regarding it as legitimate. This amounts to saying that *the risks of empowering the institution with the support that goes along with the belief that it is legitimate (in the normative sense) are worth taking*. Regarding an institution as legitimate in the normative sense, as possessing rightful authority, is therefore a double-edged sword: on the one hand, it is necessary if the institution is to provide the benefits that make it valuable; on the other, it empowers the institution and that power can be misused or abused.

The basic point, then, is that institutions can provide valuable benefits without dangerous levels of coercion only if they receive the support that comes from the pervasive belief that they exercise rightful authority, but that support can also empower the institution to act contrary to our interests. So, a judgment that an institution is legitimate in the normative sense is in effect the conclusion that the benefits the institution provides are sufficiently valuable to warrant the risks of abuse or error that empowering it by our support entail. Institutions that score well on the criteria are more likely to warrant taking the risk of empowering them with our support.

The comparative benefit condition 4 above provides a link between sociological and normative legitimacy. It specifies that an institution must provide substantial benefits relative to the noninstitutional situation if it is to be legitimate in the normative sense; but whether it can do this will depend upon whether it enjoys sociological legitimacy. If the support that is generated by the pervasive belief that the institution exercises rightful authority is necessary for satisfaction of the comparative benefit condition, then sociological legitimacy is important for normative legitimacy.[2]

Given that this is so, *it is vital for an institution to be perceived to exercise rightful authority, not just to do so*. The institutional measures I recommend

2. I am grateful to Paul Tucker for impressing upon me the importance of sociological legitimacy for normative legitimacy. However, I think he goes too far in saying that normative legitimacy is a subset of sociological legitimacy, because an institution can enjoy sociological legitimacy and yet be normatively illegitimate. That would occur if there were widespread overly optimistic false beliefs about how the institution was performing.

in this chapter are designed both to contribute directly to normative legitimacy by satisfying the conditions listed above, but also to enhance sociological legitimacy, where this is understood to be crucial for the institution operating effectively without undue recourse to coercion. What follows is a list of the chief institutional features that are needed to make the institutions responsible for pandemic policy both normatively and sociologically legitimate.

1. The rules that constitute the institution should include an explicit requirement that dissenting views should be solicited and publicly responded to on the merits *during the process of forging a policy*.

2. Once a policy is provisionally settled upon, it should be publicly announced and criticisms of it should be solicited and publicly responded to on the merits. Attempts to discredit those who voice dissenting views should be strictly prohibited; the substance of their views must be responsibly addressed. This applies as well to dissenting voices during the process of forming a policy (see 1 above).

3. Unelected powerful positions in national public health agencies should be term-limited, with prohibitions on retiring officials gaining remuneration from any entities that are affected by the operations of the institution.

4. There should be regular, impartial, periodic reviews of institutional performance, with a clear designation of accountability holders, criteria for adequate institutional performance (standards of accountability), and effective provision for imposing serious costs on responsible agents in the event of a negative evaluation.

5. All major policy decisions should be subject to a requirement of explicit, public justification, where this includes, inter alia, a non-technical presentation of the results of a thorough cost-benefit analysis, along with a way to access the information upon which the cost-benefit analysis was based. The cost-benefit analysis should not be conducted by those proposing the policy.

6. All major operations of the institution should be subject to a transparency requirement, with the presumption that there should be transparency at the time the operations are occurring. Where there are good reasons not to require contemporaneous transparency, there should be a requirement of ex-post transparency. It should not be up to the sole discretion of the institution's agents to determine

when the requirement of contemporaneous transparency may
be waived.

7. There should be legal prohibitions on political officials and agents
attempting to influence the policies of the FDA, CDC, and HHS
regarding pandemic responses. Political pressure from the Executive Branch should be strictly forbidden. Guidance for how to
insulate policy experts from political interference should be sought
from Swedish law.[3]

Each of these requirements is commonsensical, *yet none of them is currently
in place.*

Item 5, as I have already suggested, is important for both prudential
and moral reasons. From a purely prudential standpoint, the fulfillment of
this requirement provides considerable protection against official abuses
and errors and to that extent enhances the quality and accountability of
institutional decision-making. But to stop with that observation would be
to underestimate the importance of the public justification requirement.
It is morally imperative because it is a public acknowledgment of the equal
basic moral status of every person subject to the institution's policies.

A key element of the public acknowledgment of equal basic status is
the commitment to addressing all persons as reasonable, as beings who
can engage with one another on the basis of a mutual commitment to
giving and receiving reasons. To fail to offer justifications for institutional
conduct is to deny this fundamental status and instead to treat citizens as if
they were mere objects, things to be commanded, or as minors incapable of
being reasoned with. Not bearing the burden of public justification betrays
an elitist, paternalistic, and demeaning attitude toward citizens.

I have no intention of trying to justify the claim that all persons are
owed a public recognition of their status as reasoning beings. In my judgment, this is as close to a fundamental, nonderivative, moral truth as one
is likely to encounter. However, I am aware of no justification for rejecting
it that does not rely on false factual claims about supposedly profoundly
morally relevant differences among groups of human beings. For example,
defenses of caste systems and racial and gender hierarchies always rely on
unsubstantiated claims about the inferior mental or moral characteristics
of those who are to be treated as less than equal. In addition, those who

---

3. These desiderata are similar to the "principles of delegation" advocated by Paul Tucker
in his excellent book *Unelected Power: The Quest for Legitimacy in Central Banking and the
Regulatory State* (Cambridge, MA: Harvard University Press, 2018).

reject the equal basic status view typically make another error: they assume that whatever differences in intelligence or moral capacities can actually be scientifically documented are morally important enough to justify a denial of basic equality.

There are in fact three ways to argue for a strong requirement of public justifications for institutional policies. I have already distinguished the prudential argument from what might be called the fundamental argument, according to which equal respect requires justification. The third support for the public justification is provided by a highly influential contemporary moral theory or rather a family of theories called Public Reason Liberalism or Justificatory Liberalism.[4]

According to this family of views, public justification for institutional policies that rely on coercion, even if only as a last resort, is a necessary condition for institutional legitimacy in the normative sense, not just something that is instrumentally valuable as a contributor to sociological legitimacy. I do not elaborate this sort of view or defend it against those who have criticized or qualified it. I observe, however, that it may well be that it is grounded ultimately in the more fundamental commitment to treating persons as reasonable beings, creatures who are owed reasons for actions that affect them. If that is so, then it is more accurate to see the Public Reason or Justificatory Liberalism view as providing a specification, in the case of coercive institutions, of the implications of the more fundamental equal basic status view rather than as an alternative to it. In this view, the best way to ensure that the requirement that a policy is in fact justifiable to all affected by it is to provide a public justification and solicit criticisms of it.

If I were pressed to identify a single principle that undergirds most if not all of the items on the list of institutional characteristics 1–7 above, I would say it is this: institutions charged with responding to a pandemic, like all public institutions, should be structured in such a way as to provide a public expression of equal respect for persons. Doing that requires publicly justifying policies and ensuring that institutional agents are accountable to the public.

4. Among the most prominent proponents of public reason liberalism are John Rawls and Gerald Gaus. See John Rawls, *Political Liberalism* (New York: Columbia University Press, 1993), and Gerald Gaus, *The Order of Public Reason* (Cambridge: Cambridge University Press, 2011). For a more precise and shorter discussion of public reason liberalism, see Gerald Gaus, "Public Reason Liberalism," in *The Cambridge Companion to Liberalism,* edited by Steven Wall, 112–40 (Cambridge: Cambridge University Press, 2015).

ARE THESE PROPOSALS FOR INSTITUTIONAL
REFORM FEASIBLE?

Compared to the status quo, my recommendations for institutional innovations are quite demanding. The worry is that if they were implemented, it would be hard to find qualified people to occupy key institutional positions. Plausible candidates for such positions would find the institutional rules too constraining, too onerous.

My first response is simple: let's try what I recommend and then we will see whether this really is a problem. But my second response is, I think, more plausible. The requirements I propose are mainly procedural. It is therefore relatively easy for institutional agents to operate in a way that minimizes the risk that they will be unjustly penalized: they need only follow the specified procedures. Further, the requirements I propose, especially those regarding the imposition of costs for malfeasance, are to be implemented in the context of well-known and commonsensical notions of due process, where these include a distinction between culpable and nonculpable mistakes and the notion of due diligence (as opposed to omniscience).

More importantly, even if some of my suggestions are unrealistic, not feasible at present or for the foreseeable future or not compatible with attracting able persons to institutional positions, they can at least provide guidance for the direction of change. Even an approximation to fulfilling them would be a marked improvement over the status quo.

HOW ELITIST-PATERNALISTIC BEHAVIOR CREATES A SOCIAL
EXPERIENCE THAT SEEMS TO CONFIRM ITS ASSUMPTIONS

I conclude this chapter with an observation about what tends to happen when the requirement of public justification is not satisfied. Citizens are treated as if they were incapable of being convinced to support institutional policy on the basis of reasons they can appreciate. Once institutional agents regard citizens in this way, they are likely to deprive them of the information and opportunities required for engagement on the basis of reasons. In other words, acting on the presumption that citizens are not owed justifications for public policies because they are not up to the task can become a self-fulfilling prophecy.

Here an analogy with another case of elitist-paternalistic behavior, noted earlier, is illustrative. Physicians in neonatal care units routinely excluded parents from decision-making regarding the care of their severely impaired newborns, and did not share important information with them. They thereby created a situation that seemed to confirm their low estimate of the parents' capacities for decision-making and more generally for participation in an exchange of reasons regarding treatment decisions.

Similarly, if institutional agents are accustomed to regarding ordinary citizens as incompetent to judge the quality of institutional policies, and as not owed justifications because of the institutional agents' inflated understandings of their own expertise, they will deprive them of the information and opportunities for learning that they need if they are to operate as reasonable beings. Put most simply, elitist-paternalistic behavior tends to create an experience that seems to justify it. Whether people can participate as equals in the exchange of reasons can depend upon whether those in power treat them as being capable of such participation.

FIVE

The Need for International
Institutional Innovation

The international response to COVID-19 has been disappointing. Wealthy countries have hoarded vaccines far in excess of their needs and signed contracts with vaccine suppliers stipulating that they cannot distribute their surpluses to other countries. While wealthy countries and medical supply companies, including vaccine producers, have publicly acknowledged that they ought to do something to alleviate the plight of under-resourced countries, their efforts have been both uncoordinated and inadequate. As was noted in Chapter One, several international entities, including WHO, Gavi, and COVAX have done something to remedy these deficiencies, but not nearly enough.[1]

In this chapter I first develop an ethical-conceptual framework and then use it to ground a proposal for a new international institution designed to provide a more effective response to the plight of poorer countries in the face of a pandemic. I begin by drawing out the moral implications of the assumption that a pandemic is a global health emergency, a situation

---

1. Gavi, the Vaccine Alliance is an international organization that was dedicated initially to improving access to new and underused vaccines for children living in the world's poorest countries. During the COVID-19 epidemic it expanded its role to facilitate access to COVID-19 vaccines. COVID-19 Vaccines Global Access, abbreviated as COVAX, is a global effort to provide equitable access to COVID-19 vaccines.

in which people in many countries are in need of rapid interventions to prevent them from suffering death or serious harms.

THE DUTY TO RESCUE

Emergencies have these characteristics: there is a serious threat of imminent serious harm, the timing of the occurrence of the threat was unpredictable, and averting the harm requires rapid action. If a potential harm is imminent and very serious, we can say that those who will suffer the harm, unless it is averted, are in need of rescue.[2] Timely provision of ventilators, for example, could count as rescue in the context of a pandemic, as could the provision of intensive care specialists and life-saving therapeutics.

The duty to rescue is not the only relevant basic duty implicated in a global pandemic. There is also a duty to prevent foreseeable harms due to a pandemic when these harms are not imminent, as they are in rescue situations. Although I focus on the duty to rescue, much of what I say applies as well to the duty to prevent serious harms.

My aim in this chapter is twofold: first, to show that in the context of a pandemic that constitutes an emergency, fulfilling the duty to rescue and more generally the duty to mitigate or prevent serious harms to innocent people requires institutional innovation at the international level; and second, to begin to characterize the key features of the needed international institution. My investigation might be framed using the notion of the duty of Samaritanism rather than that of rescue: both convey the idea of an individual or collective being in a position to render the aid needed to avert serious harm to another.

I argue that in preparation for another global health emergency, including another pandemic, governments, civil society organizations, and pharmaceutical companies have a duty of justice to work together to create a treaty-based institution that will perfect imperfect duties to rescue and more generally to prevent and mitigate serious harms. Before I can make the case for this institutional innovation, it is first necessary to develop an account of the duty to rescue. Having done that, I then show how two polar political views, extreme cosmopolitanism and extreme nationalism, understand the duty to rescue. I then argue that neither provides a

2. I have argued elsewhere that the emergency framing is perilous unless one is careful to do two things: ask what the scope of the emergency is (who exactly is at high risk for serious harm) and reevaluate over time whether the emergency exists and, if so, whether its scope has changed ("Learning from Flawed Responses to the Covid-19 Pandemic," *Social Philosophy & Policy*, forthcoming).

plausible answer to a fundamental question: What are the proper scope and limits of national partiality in a global health emergency? Articulating the flaws of these two views will take us some distance toward understanding the contours of the duties that are in need of being perfected by institutionalization.

Cosmopolitans have an expansive conception of the duty to rescue and more generally of the duty to prevent serious harms to innocent people; moral nationalists have a highly constrained conception of it. Moral cosmopolitans of the most extreme sort believe that all institutions, including national ones—and even under emergency conditions—should treat all persons as being worthy of equal consideration. Extreme nationalists, in contrast, believe that national institutions are morally permitted if not obligated to show exclusive concern for a country's own citizens, at least when it comes to positive duties, including duties of rescue. (Even the most extreme nationalists, at least if they are in the broadly liberal camp, acknowledge that national partiality is limited by negative duties toward foreigners, including duties not to kill them, enslave them, or expropriate their territories.)

Thomas Pogge is a highly influential cosmopolitan, while David Miller is in my judgment the most articulate representative of the nationalist view.[3] Below I explore the implications of their respective positions for how the duty to rescue bears on the question of the proper scope and limits of national partiality in a global health emergency such as the current COVID-19 pandemic. First, it is necessary to clarify the duty to rescue in a way that is neutral as to the differences between moral cosmopolitans and moral nationalists. My conclusions also apply more generally to the duty to prevent and mitigate serious harms, whether or not they are imminent.

Philosophers usually discuss the duty to rescue by focusing on a highly simplified, extreme case—a case of easy rescue of one victim by one rescuer. You see a child drowning in a shallow pond. You alone can save the child's life and you can do so without excessive cost to yourself. Cosmopolitans like Pogge and nationalists like Miller both hold that you have a duty to save the child and that that it is a duty of justice—that you owe the duty to the child or, to put the same point differently, that she has a right to your aid and will be wronged by you if you fail to provide it.

3. See Thomas Pogge, *World Poverty and Human Rights* (Cambridge: Polity Press, 2002) and David Miller, *National Responsibility and Global Justice* (Oxford: Oxford University Press, 2012).

Further, both cosmopolitans and nationalists can acknowledge that the duty to rescue applies more broadly; that it is not limited to cases where the potential rescuer is in close physical proximity to the person in peril. Yet there is a difference as to how the two camps understand the duty in such cases. Cosmopolitans believe that we have *duties of justice* to render aid to persons in severely disadvantaged or perilous circumstances even if they are "distant strangers"—that is, they are far away, are not our fellow citizens, and we have no special relationship to them. Nationalists deny that we have duties of justice to rescue distant strangers; instead, they believe we only have *duties of beneficence* (or charity or humanity). To appreciate the significance of these contrasting characterizations of the duty to rescue distant strangers, we need to get clear on the distinction between duties of justice and duties of beneficence (or charity or humanity).

Duties of justice are traditionally said to be perfect duties, which means they are directed duties, owed to someone in particular; and that they have determinate content, where this includes a clear specification of what the duty-bearer must do to fulfill the duty. Duties of beneficence, in contrast, are imperfect duties: they are not owed to any one in particular and they are indeterminate in the sense of allowing the duty-bearer discretion as to whom to aid, when to provide, and what form of aid to render. Further, duties of justice are thought to be enforceable; duties of beneficence are not.

Extreme Nationalism

Let us first consider Miller's view, exploring its implications for the scope and limits of national partiality in a global health emergency such as a pandemic. According to Miller, we have a perfect duty of rescue, a duty of justice, a determinate duty owed to the person in peril, only when the following three conditions are satisfied—and it so happens that they are typically only satisfied in cases where the potential rescuer is in close physical proximity to the person in peril.

Suppose that I am the potential rescuer and you are the person in peril. First, I must be uniquely positioned to save you; second, we must encounter each other in such a way that there is a mutual recognition that your safety depends uniquely on me; and third, the encounter must be within the bounds of my "personal space," a physical domain in which I can exercise considerable control and therefore within which I have significant responsibilities. Since Miller thinks these conditions are generally satisfied only when the potential rescuer and the one in need of rescue are in close proximity, he is committed to the view that we do not have duties of justice to citizens of other countries to help them avoid death and serious injury due to a global pandemic.

This is where Miller leaves us: with only imperfect duties to help foreigners in peril. And this, in my judgment, is a morally untenable location. That is because imperfect duties have a number of imperfections. First, the discretion that characterizes imperfect duties permits moral laxity. One is morally lax if, over an extended period of time, one fails to take serious steps toward achieving a goal one views oneself as morally committed to. In the case of an imperfect duty to rescue, one may be tempted to rationalize doing nothing by consoling oneself with the thought that "Well, I'll do something at some point, for some of those people in peril—and there will always be plenty of such people." Second, due to their inherent vagueness as to how much aid to provide to whom and in what form, imperfect duties are subject to disagreement among those who acknowledge that they have the duty. Such disagreement has two unfortunate consequences: it will be difficult to achieve any consensus on how to evaluate the behavior of the relevant agents and thus difficult for them to hold each other accountable. Third, even if agents do not succumb to moral laxity and strive to fulfill their duties in the absence of accountability, their efforts are likely to be uncoordinated, with the result that there will be both gaps and redundancies in aid.

Fourth, where duties are imperfect, agents may rationalize not acting because they lack assurance that others will act appropriately: they may be unwilling to bear the costs of providing aid if they think others similarly situated are not bearing those costs. This is a feature of the lack of enforceability and, more broadly, the lack of accountability that is due to the indeterminacy of the duties. Fifth, where effective aid requires contributions by many parties, the free-rider problem may undercut successful collective action. Each party may reason that either enough others will contribute to achieve success in achieving some particular goal or they will not, regardless of whether she contributes. She may tell herself that it will be better, morally, if she only provides aid independently, not as part of a collective effort.

Enforcement can solve such collective action problems, but if imperfect duties are unenforceable, that option is not available. The point is that, in some cases, effective aid can only be rendered through a collective effort because it depends on some threshold of contributions being reached that is beyond the resources of any particular individual. If individuals, either because of the free-rider problem or the assurance problem, do not contribute to such collective aid projects and engage only in independent aid provision, the result may be extremely inefficient.

In brief, in the real world, when it comes to quite imperfect creatures like us, relying solely on imperfect duties to rescue distant strangers in peril is predictably suboptimal from a moral point of view: moral underperformance is virtually guaranteed.

My main worry about Miller's view is that he ends his analysis with an implicit acceptance of a defective moral status quo and fails to consider how a better situation might be achieved. In brief, he fails to consider the fact that *we can work together to create institutions that perfect imperfect duties*—and that failure to do so is a moral fault. Or, to put it differently, he does not consider the possibility that there is a duty to prevent the predictable failures that result from relying only on imperfect duties to rescue distant foreigners. I argue that we do have such a duty and then argue that it is a duty of justice.

How can institutions perfect imperfect duties? They can (1) identify specific duty-bearers and rights-holders (2) distribute the costs of rescuing large numbers of people in a fair manner, and (3) include mechanisms for compliance with the duties they specify, either through the threat of penalties for noncompliance or rewards for compliance. Effective measures for compliance can prevent both the free-rider and assurance problems from stymying concerted efforts to provide aid and they can prevent moral laxness. Because they are both determinate and enforceable, perfect duties facilitate accountability: agents can be evaluated and either rewarded or penalized for failing to act on their professed moral commitments. The vagueness of imperfect duties, in contrast, makes accountability extremely difficult if not impossible.

This is not merely a possibility; it actually occurs. The modern welfare state is a prime example of an institution that improves our moral situation by perfecting imperfect duties. There are in fact many cases where institutions improve moral performance relative to the noninstitutional situation. They do this by changing incentives and more specifically by providing incentives that counteract moral underperformance. For example, where there are clear, justiciable, and well-enforced property rights, with determinate correlative duties, people are better able to respect other individual's claims to various objects; and opportunities for wrongful takings will be reduced. Where the law approximates key elements of the rule of law, unscrupulous government officials are less able to abuse the power of the law. The general point is that institutions can better enable us to act on our moral commitments; the particular point is that this applies to the commitment to the well-being of others that underpins the duty to rescue in the context of a pandemic.

If we have good moral reasons to rescue people in peril, then we ought to ensure that we are effective in rendering aid. Being committed to their safety means that we should not accept a situation in which aid will either not be forthcoming or will be inadequate, or will be so seriously uncoordinated that some aid is wasted by being superfluous and some people in need will not receive it. If we can improve the moral status quo by working together to create institutions that, by perfecting imperfect duties of rescue, will better achieve the goal of preventing imminent serious harms, we ought morally to do so.

An analogy may help drive this basic point home. Suppose that I regularly encounter children drowning in a pond near my home, but am not able to rescue many of them because the pond is deep, they are typically far from the shore, and I am not a strong swimmer. I am able to save some of them, the ones that happen to be near to shore, but not most. So, I direct my efforts only to those who are close enough to shore that I can reach them, given my limited skills as a swimmer.

But now suppose that I have in my possession simple instructions for building a boat that will enable me to rescue any child in peril and suppose also that I have all the necessary materials or can easily get them. I also have neighbors I can call upon to help me build the rescue boat. Surely, if I really care about saving lives, I will not rest content with a situation where my rescue efforts are so far from optimal. Instead, I will rightly feel obligated to increase the efficacy of my efforts by cooperating with my neighbors to construct a rescue boat, so long as I can do so without excessive costs.

Similarly, if we can construct institutions that will greatly increase the efficacy of our efforts to help foreigners imperiled by a pandemic, and we can do so without excessive costs to ourselves, we ought to do so. Moral consistency—indeed, integrity—requires that we do so. Notice that this conclusion applies not only to rescue, where harm is imminent, but also to prevention, where it is not.

The Moral Necessity of Institutionalizing Duties of Justice, Not Just Duties of Beneficence

My strategy has been to begin to make the case for institutional innovation in preparation for the next pandemic by starting with a premise that even the most extreme anti-cosmopolitans can accept: that there is a duty of beneficence to prevent and mitigate serious harms to distant strangers. I show that the need for institutional innovation also applies if one assumes there is a duty of justice to prevent and mitigate serious harms to distant strangers.

This conclusion seems counterintuitive if one assumes that all duties of justice are perfect duties, where this means that they are all *both* undirected *and* determinate in content, that is, specific with respect to what is required of the duty-bearer. But that assumption, I show, is unwarranted. Some duties of justice, including the duty of wealthy countries to prevent and mitigate serious harms to persons in poor countries, have only one of the two features that are said to characterize imperfect duties, namely, indeterminacy of content, while possessing one of the distinguishing features of perfect duties, namely, directedness. The more general point is that some duties of justice are quite unlike the duty to fulfill a promise, which is perfect in both respects, that is, directed and determinate in content. The failure to appreciate this fact may be due to taking the case of promising as paradigmatic of duties of justice.

In the case of the duty to prevent and mitigate serious harms due to a pandemic, there are several sources of indeterminacy as to exactly what is required of the duty-bearers. First, the duty by itself sets no priorities, yet even the resources of wealthy countries are limited and may not allow for helping all of those in peril. One needs to know whom to help first and who should get the most aid. Second, although whatever actions are to be taken to avert serious harms to those in poor countries may be constrained by some degree of partiality toward co-nationals, there is much honest disagreement about how robust this constraint is. Third, the duty to prevent and mitigate serious harms is presumably subject to a "no excessive cost" proviso; but what counts as an excessive cost may depend in part on what cost others are bearing.

For example, one country bearing disproportionately greater costs because others were not acting appropriately might be either unfair in itself or might put the more generous country at a competitive disadvantage vis-à-vis those bearing lesser costs. In the absence of institutions to determine what counts as a fair distribution of costs, duty-bearers may not be able to determine what counts as excessive costs; and until they know that they will not know what exactly is required of them. Finally, without an institution to coordinate efforts on the basis of the best information available, even conscientious government officials may not know how to provide aid in a reasonably effective and efficient manner.

The key point here is that some duties of justice are "half perfect," having only the indeterminacy of content feature but not the non-directedness feature. This applies to the duty to respect other people's property. Prior to institutional specification of the content of the right to property, one may know that others have property rights and know that some acts will clearly violate them, but the boundaries of the protections they are entitled to may be unclear. Further, there may be no one uniquely correct specification of the complex content of the right to property that is valid for all contexts. Institutional specification is needed, even if the duty in question is a duty of justice.

So, even if duties of justice are unlike imperfect duties of beneficence in that they are directed, they can in some cases share the other feature of imperfect duties, indeterminacy of content. One can know that one ought, as a matter of justice, help prevent and mitigate serious harms to distant strangers and to respect the property rights of others, but not know exactly how to proceed in order to fulfill the duty in a reasonable and responsible manner.

This indeterminacy of content in the case of the duty to prevent serious harms, even when it is considered to be a duty of justice, facilitates the moral underperformance we encountered earlier in the world in which only the duty of beneficence existed. It encourages moral laxity, bias in the provision of aid, and inefficient discoordination. To rest content with these deficiencies when they can be reduced or eliminated is itself a moral fault.

It seems clear, then, that under circumstances like those we now find ourselves in the midst of a global pandemic, we have a duty to work together to construct institutions that will enable us to act more effectively on our moral commitments by perfecting imperfect duties of rescue and more generally duties to prevent and mitigate serious harms, whether they are imminent or not. The only question is the status of those duties: are they duties of justice or duties of beneficence (or charity or humanity)? If we fail to work together to construct the needed institutions, do we wrong those who will perish because we failed to do so? Can they rightly say that we wronged them?

Here John Rawls's notion of a natural duty of justice is helpful.[4] His highly plausible claim is that, out of recognition of the basic moral equality of all persons, that is, to show proper respect and concern for all persons,

---

4. John Rawls, *A Theory of Justice: Revised Edition* (Cambridge, MA: Harvard University Press / Belknap Press, 1971, 1999): 98–101.

we ought to cooperate to create conditions in which they will enjoy the benefits of justice. This is not a new idea. Kant thought that there is a fundamental duty to create conditions in which we can relate to others in a just way. Hobbes could be interpreted as holding that the worst thing about the state of nature is that there is no justice there.

It is a commonplace that justice means giving each person her due. Following Kant and Rawls, my suggestion is that giving each person her due means, inter alia, establishing conditions in which there are clear duties of justice, if doing that is what is needed to secure their fundamental interests, including their interests in survival. In other words, I think the duty to work together to create institutions that perfect imperfect duties is a duty of justice. I think we wrong people if we fail to try to construct institutions that will perfect imperfect duties when doing so is vital for their very survival and we can do this without excessive costs to ourselves. I think that resting content with imperfect duties in such cases exhibits such a serious disregard for the welfare and freedom of those in peril as to constitute a failure to acknowledge their basic equal moral status as persons and that this is to wrong them, to fail to accord them what is their due.

But it might be replied that the duty to construct institutions to perfect imperfect duties is itself very abstract and indeterminate. Therefore, it cannot qualify as a perfect duty and hence cannot be a duty of justice.

I would argue that at present that is not so. We have good reason to believe there will be another pandemic and we cannot be confident that it will only occur so far in the future that we need do nothing now to prepare for it. Consequently, there is something very specific that wealthier countries, pharmaceutical companies, and health-related civil society organizations ought to do *now*, namely, begin the process of building an institution to create a fair distribution of effectively incentivized, directed duties to ensure that those most endangered by the next global health crisis receive relief. Because it is unclear how long it will take to build the needed institutions, it is imperative to start now. One cannot plausibly say: "Oh, well, we'll do something, sometime." This would be like saying, "Oh, well, someday I'll build a boat to rescue children farther out in the pond" when a child may be drowning in the middle of the lake tomorrow.

In the current pandemic, we have seen the moral failures that result from the lack of institutions that would perfect imperfect duties—institutions that would identify duty bearers, direct their duties toward specific recipients of aid, fairly distribute the duties so that no one bears unacceptably high or disproportionate costs in fulfilling their duties, and provides effective incentives for compliance with the assigned duties. Governments of wealthy countries and leaders of pharmaceutical companies have for the most part acknowledged that they ought to do *something* to ensure that poor countries have access to vaccines and other medical resources, but little has been done.

When duties are left imperfect, it is all but impossible to hold governments or pharmaceutical companies to account. Imperfect duties are too indeterminate and allow the duty-bearer too much discretion to make accountability feasible. Matters change dramatically when we can point to determinate, directed duties and ask whether they are being fulfilled.

Whether institutions that can perfect duties of rescue in a global pandemic can be constructed will depend crucially on the cooperation of governments and pharmaceutical companies. The public ought to mobilize to hold them accountable for helping to create conditions in which they can be held accountable. Acting alone, members of the public may have little power, but civil society organizations can mobilize and focus public opinion in ways that governments and pharmaceutical companies may find it difficult to ignore. In my judgment, under present conditions, the duty to construct institutions that will enable us to perfect imperfect duties in anticipation of the next pandemic is sufficiently determinate to guide action. And this duty is directed both in the sense that we know who the major contributors should be and who will be the most in need of aid— namely, the already disadvantaged.

A Dynamic Conception of Morality

My criticism of Miller can now be recast in general terms that have broad implications for moral philosophy. I reject his implicit and insupportable assumption that the boundaries of justice are fixed and more specifically that the duty to rescue, as a duty of justice, cannot extend to rescuing distant strangers.[5] If, as his analysis implies, under present conditions there are only imperfect duties, not duties of justice to prevent massive imminent harms to foreigners when we can do so without serious cost to ourselves, then the proper response is not to acquiesce in this morally deficient situation but to change it. I have argued that the duty to perfect imperfect duties in this case is a duty of justice. Whether that is so or not is irrelevant, however, to my dissatisfaction with where Miller's analysis leaves us. He takes the moral landscape as fixed, not recognizing that we can and ought to change it.

5. Allen Buchanan, "Justice and Charity," *Ethics* 97 no. 3 (1987): 558–75.

Unfortunately, I think this static view of morality—in this case the assumption that the boundary between justice, on the one hand, and beneficence (or charity or humanity), on the other, is forever fixed—is all too common in contemporary moral philosophy.[6] The problem with the static view is that it underestimates the power of human beings to transform their moral predicament and thereby erects an obstacle to moral progress. If we assume the static viewpoint, we can only wring our hands in response to some of the worst deficiencies of responses to the current pandemic; we will not be in a position to see that we can do better next time around.

I conclude, then, that Miller has not vindicated an extreme nationalist position; he has given us no good reason to think that the duty of rescue cannot be invoked to ground a policy of restricting national partiality for the sake of rescuing distant strangers, as a matter of justice. More specifically, he has not shown that rich countries suffering relatively low mortality and morbidity from the pandemic have no obligations of justice to provide aid to countries where the pandemic is much more lethal and that lack the resources for limiting its lethality. My aim, however, is not to criticize Miller, but to expose the shortcomings of any extreme nationalist view on duties of rescue in a pandemic.

Extreme Cosmopolitanism

I now turn to an analysis of Pogge's view, as perhaps the most developed and prominent instance of an extreme cosmopolitan view that has clear implications for how we ought to frame our response to a global pandemic. He argues that citizens of wealthy countries have duties of justice to combat poverty and disease in poor countries, not just in the special case of pandemics, but on an ongoing basis, because they are morally responsible for the disadvantaged positions the people of those countries occupy and that make them especially vulnerable to disease. Pogge thinks we are responsible for their disadvantaged position and its negative health consequences because we have caused the harms they suffer by participating in (and benefitting from) an unjust international order. Pogge does not frame his argument in terms of the duty to rescue. Nonetheless, it will be fruitful to construe it that way, since his approach to helping the world's most disadvantaged people can accommodate the idea that in some cases their plight is so dire that the notion of rescue applies.

6. For an argument to show that the boundaries of justice are not fixed, see Buchanan, "Justice and Charity."

In the case at hand, Pogge might well argue that most if not all countries that cannot afford vaccines are in this predicament because their economic development has been impeded by certain features of the international order, features that facilitate destructive, exploitive behavior on the part of both their own governments and powerful states and corporations. Instead of relying on a duty of rescue understood as a positive duty, or more generally, on a duty to prevent dire harm, whether imminent or not, Pogge opts for the idea of a duty of justice to mitigate harms for which we are responsible because we have caused them.

I find this approach to be both problematic and unnecessarily indirect. Pogge develops it because he thinks it is less controversial to argue for relieving the plight of the world's worst off people from the premise that there is a duty not to harm, a negative duty, than from the premise that there is a positive duty, more specifically a duty to prevent harms one has not caused and is not in any way responsible for. Whether Pogge is right in assuming that more people will in fact acknowledge a negative rather than a positive duty is an empirical matter on which I choose not to speculate. But I think it is clear that Pogge's argument for why those in wealthier countries have a duty of justice to repair the damage of the international system they supposedly support and are causally implicated in is dubious. Opting for a duty not to harm in this case turns out to be a lot more costly in terms of argumentative cogency than Pogge assumes.

Pogge's approach is problematic for at least two reasons: first, it is far from clear that by merely acquiescing and/or benefitting from the unjust international order one is causing the harm it produces or is for some other reason responsible for that harm. Even if it could be established that you and I are making some causal contribution, it is presumably so miniscule as to be incapable of grounding any significant obligation. Second, Pogge overestimates the power of ordinary citizens to control their country's policies—in this case, to achieve a fundamental reform of the international order or, failing that, to facilitate a massive transfer of resources from the rich to the poor. Further, if we lack this control, then it is all the more implausible to say either that we are causing the harms inflicted by that order or that we are responsible for them.

In addition, Pogge's approach is unnecessarily indirect because it assumes that one must first establish causal responsibility for a harm in order to show that one has a duty of justice to prevent that harm. That, in effect, is simply to deny that any duty of rescue is a duty of justice, including the duty to save the child in the pond. That is an extremely implausible view. One needn't show that a person is responsible for the child being in the pond in order to show that that person has a duty of justice to rescue the child.

My framing of the need to act in a global emergency avoids both the drawbacks of Pogge's view and the disturbing complacency of Miller's. My argument for why, as a matter of justice, we ought to work together to create institutions that will extend the domain of justice and not rest content with imperfect duties does not assume, as Pogge's argument does, that we are obligated, as a matter of justice, only for mitigating those harms we ourselves cause. On my view, it is not necessary to show that we are responsible in any way, either directly or indirectly, for the harms we have a duty of justice to work together to create conditions in which we can effectively prevent it.

A Positive Cosmopolitan Duty

Given the problems of Pogge's brand of cosmopolitanism, it is worth considering whether a cosmopolitan account of the duty to rescue might be developed on the basis of a positive duty to aid, more specifically a duty to prevent serious harms to innocent persons. The straightforward idea here would be that it is unnecessary to show that the better off have somehow caused the special vulnerability of the worst off to the damage due to a pandemic. Instead, they have a duty to prevent and mitigate from serious, pandemic-caused harms simply as a matter of recognizing the equal worth of all persons. In its extreme form, this cosmopolitan view denies that any national partiality is justified: aid should be rendered on the basis of need, regardless of boundaries.

I assess this version of cosmopolitanism indirectly, by considering the limitations of three arguments for national partiality. The upshot of my analysis is that although these three arguments do not vindicate extreme nationalism, they do suffice to discredit extreme cosmopolitanism, including versions of that view that, unlike Pogge's account, rely on a positive duty. One advantage of this strategy is that my assessments apply to both the duty to rescue and the duty to prevent and mitigate non-imminent pandemic-caused harms.

The three arguments for extreme national priority are (1) the argument from the division of labor, (2) the argument from special obligations, and (3) the argument from local knowledge. Let us consider each in turn.

It is a fact about our world that there is no world government and that if justice and welfare are to be achieved it will be largely within and partly through the efforts of states. Given the lack of a world government and the greater resources and capacities of states relative to other institutions, it makes sense to acknowledge a division of labor, with states having the chief responsibility for the freedom and welfare of those within their jurisdiction. But if states are to fulfill this role it is proper that they should show partiality to their own citizens—after all, the responsibility for securing the freedom and welfare of those people rests on the shoulders of their state.

This first argument suffices to show that states may show *some* partiality to their own citizens in a global emergency such as the current pandemic. But it falls short of justifying the extreme partiality that the wealthier countries have in fact exhibited. That is because the argument is subject to two important limitations. The first and most obvious is that not all countries have the resources or the government leadership to discharge the burden of securing the welfare and freedom of their citizens without external help. This simple fact is of extreme importance in the current pandemic because it is well documented that pandemics are usually most damaging in poorer countries. Such countries have more vulnerable populations due to poor medical care, nutrition, sanitation, and housing prior to the pandemic and because they have fewer resources for mitigating the damage caused by the pandemic.

The second limitation on the division of labor argument for national partiality is that wealthy countries have surplus capacity when it comes to responding effectively to a pandemic like the one we are now experiencing. They can reduce the risk of the pandemic to their own citizens to reasonable levels, compatible with their fiduciary duties to them, and still have resources to bestow on countries that will suffer much greater harm if they do not receive external aid. When one combines the fact that some countries cannot achieve a reasonable response to the pandemic on their own with the fact that some countries have surplus capacity and resources, the inescapable conclusion is that the division of labor argument does not establish the conclusion that countries may exercise unrestrained partiality.

To drive home this point it is necessary to explain what counts as surplus capacity and resources. Surplus here means in excess of what is *adequate*, not what is *optimal* from the standpoint of reducing COVID-19 infection or medical or economic damage due to infections. To assume the latter would be to make the fundamental errors noted earlier: to ignore the marginal costs of risk reduction—including the costs to others who will be deprived of resources used for additional increments of risk reduction—and to think that the proper goal is to reduce the risk to as near to zero as possible.[7]

As noted earlier, in the early stages of a global health threat, when there is great uncertainty as to just how bad things may get, state leaders, in honoring their special fiduciary obligations to their own citizens are permitted act with extreme partiality. In other words, under these conditions it is appropriate for leaders and the public to employ the emergency framing and to act on the assumption that national partiality is permitted. But once it becomes clear that the situation for those in wealthy countries is not so dire—and indeed that it is no longer right to call it an emergency—such extreme partiality is no longer justified.

In my judgment, it became clear quite some time ago that the risks posed to citizens of most of the wealthier countries was not so severe, relative to the resources those countries possess, that their leaders should disregard the far greater needs of people who don't happen to be their fellow citizens. And, as I also suggested earlier, it is simply incredible to assume that we are still in an emergency if morbidity and mortality from COVID-19 reach levels close to that of a normal or even somewhat unusually severe flu season.

The key point here is that once we have gotten past the extreme uncertainty of the initial situation, what a country regards as an acceptable level of resource expenditure to protect its own citizens should not only avoid the hysteria of trying to reduce harm to zero, but should also take into account the proportion between the harm to its own citizens that can be averted by additional risk reduction measures and the harm that foreigners will suffer if they do not have access to those resources.

Let me hasten to add that I am not advocating significant limitations on national partiality in all circumstances. I am willing to take seriously the possibility that if we faced a pandemic that was both more easily transmitted than COVID-19 and also had a much, much greater case morbidity

7. As I argued in an earlier chapter, unfortunately some public health experts seem to have convinced U.S. government leaders that the goal is to stop or reduce as much as possible the spread of COVID-19—without regard to the economic, psychosocial, and other costs of doing so. That goal is morally untenable for two reasons: first, even from the standpoint of an exclusive focus on the well-being of Americans, it is wrong to ignore the costs of reducing the harms caused by COVID-19; second, continuing to pursue the goal of stopping the spread of the virus beyond the point at which the risk caused by infection to Americans is tolerable is most likely to result in this wealthy country not doing enough to help people in greater need in poorer countries. There is one more negative consequence of the obsession with stopping the spread of the virus: it obscures a hard moral question, namely, how much cost should the vast majority who are not at risk of death or serious damage from COVID-19 bear to try to protect a tiny minority at high risk.

rate—say 40 percent—it would be a kind of lifeboat ethics situation in which extreme, virtually unlimited national partiality would be justified. Or, I should say, such extreme partiality would be justified until the emergency had subsided. In other words, in a much more lethal pandemic than the one we are now experiencing, national partiality might trump the triage principle and negate the duty to rescue foreigners. The point is simply that we in the wealthier countries are nowhere near that extreme situation now, though our leaders are acting as if we were.

It is also worth pointing out that the argument from the division of labor features a gaping logical gap: from the premise that there is no world government it does not follow that each country should be responsible for the health needs of its citizens. That is because the only alternatives are not a world government or exclusive reliance on self-help. A third alternative is to develop specific international institutions to convert imperfect duties of rescue to perfect duties of justice. Further, the institutional innovation could be quite specific and limited: its mission could be restricted to responding equitably and effectively to global pandemics. Once we understand the flaws of the division of labor argument it becomes clear that we should not succumb to the following fallacy: justifying refusal to cooperate to construct international institutions to create a duty to rescue as a duty of justice on the grounds that it conflicts with national partiality and then justifying national partiality on the grounds that each nation must look out for itself exclusively because of the lack of international institutions.

The second argument, for national partiality, is simple: on the whole, the citizens of a country are in ongoing relationships of interdependence that are denser than their relations with foreigners. Special relationships generate special obligations here (as they do in families and friendships). The state, as the agent of the people, should facilitate the fulfillment of those obligations. Among those obligations are those of aid in times of danger. So, because of the special relationships among co-nationals and the special obligations they generate, it is appropriate for the state to exhibit national partiality in the face of a pandemic.

The problem with this second argument is, that like the argument from the division of labor, it only shows that some partiality, in some circumstances, is warranted, without either acknowledging or illuminating the moral limits of partiality. This becomes clear when we probe the analogy that proponents of the argument almost invariably use: that of the family or a friendship. If I am a wealthy person and there are many people who are not my friends or family who are in desperate need, then I can show proper partiality to those near and dear to me and still do something significant for the worst off. Showing proper partiality to my son doesn't mean giving him a Mercedes rather than a Chevrolet, especially if the difference between what a Mercedes costs and a Chevrolet costs would save the life of someone who doesn't happen to be my son. Similarly, proper partiality toward American citizens does not mean spending all the money that might reduce the risk of COVID-19 infection for all of them, rather than focusing on the most vulnerable of them.

The third argument, which attempts to ground national partiality in the superiority of local knowledge, is even flimsier than the preceding two—if considered as an argument for extreme, virtually unlimited partiality. Yes, it is true that local knowledge is often superior. But that is not always true when it comes to public health knowledge. Some countries are so poor that they lack not only a decent medical infrastructure but also decent information infrastructure, especially for information relevant to responding effectively to a pandemic. But even where local knowledge is superior, this does not rule out external aid; it only rules out external aid that ignores rather than partners with people on the ground to take advantage of local knowledge.

An assessment of the three arguments for national partiality yields this conclusion, then: at best they show that some national partiality is justified in some circumstances and that consequently extreme cosmopolitanism, which denies the permissibility of any national partiality whatsoever, is untenable. But they do not establish extreme national partiality. This means that the duties that are to be institutionalized will reflect a rejection of both extreme cosmopolitanism and extreme nationalism. In this essay I do not have the space to say more about the contours of the duties to be institutionalized, but instead now proceed to outline what the institution should look like. Doing so will, I hope, help start the process of developing a moral coordination point that can lend sufficient determinacy to the duty to create the institution so as to vindicate my claim that there is such a duty and that it is already or soon could be determinate enough to be taken seriously.

INSTITUTIONAL DESIGN

My chief conclusion in this chapter so far has been that there is a need for international institutional innovation to ensure a more effective, efficient and ethical response to a future pandemic X than was seen in the COVID pandemic. We need such innovation regardless of whether (as cosmopolitans think) the duty to rescue distant strangers is a duty of justice or (as nationalists think) a duty of beneficence. I have also argued that the duty to help create the needed institution will itself remain unhelpfully indeterminate without a normative coordination point, at least an outline of the main features the institution should possess. In this part, I begin the task of supplying that.

CREATION OR MODIFICATION?

Should it be a new institution or a modification of an existing one? There are existing three candidates for modification: WHO, Gavi, and COVAX. In my judgment, each is sufficiently problematic that building on it would be inadvisable.

WHO has suffered a loss of sociological legitimacy that will make it difficult for it to take on the more ambitious mission of perfecting imperfect duties of rescue in a pandemic. In particular, it has proved unable to stand up to China in demanding timely information concerning the origins and early spread of COVID-19, and is more generally unable to act effectively in the face of political pressure from member states, especially the most powerful of these. It has also been unable or unwilling to work well with pharmaceutical companies.

Gavi has operated with a seriously defective rationing system that ignores differences in need among vaccine recipient countries. In addition, its policies are unduly influenced by the preferences of one major donor, the Gates Foundation.

COVAX has not achieved its vaccine distribution goal—only 5 percent of the projected 2 billion doses—and the overall distribution achieved has been grossly inequitable (90 percent to the richest G20 countries). In addition, there have been justifiable complaints of lack of transparency.[8]

Given these problems, there is much to be said for creating a new institution, one that will not inherit the credibility deficits that would be entailed by building on any or all three of these entities. So let us now consider, in broad outline, what a new institution should look like.

KEY MORAL DESIDERATA

First, there is a need for principles and mechanisms for the distribution to poorer countries of vaccines and other medical supplies needed in a pandemic, compatible with fair rationing of these resources within countries.

---

8. Katerini Tagmatarchi Storeng, Antoine de Bengy Puyvallée, and Felix Stein, "COVAX and the Rise of the 'Super Public Private Partnership' for Global Health," *Global Public Health* (2021): 2.

Second, the institution should at least approximate a fair distribution of the costs of providing aid, in part by a progressive schedule of contributions, with richer countries paying more. Third, the institution should be structured in such a way as to guarantee meaningful participation by the beneficiaries of aid, especially with regard to the development of standards for accountability.

STRUCTURAL-PROCEDURAL DESIDERATA

1. The design of the institution should exemplify incentive compatibility with regard to joining, continued participation, and general institutional functioning.

2. The institution should also be designed and presented to publics in such a fashion as to achieve sociological legitimacy, without which it will be unlikely to function successfully. Institutional agents should be formally required to provide public justifications for major policy decisions, where this includes presentation of the results of cost-benefit analysis and disclosure of the publicly accessible information on which the analysis was based.

3. Both during the policy formation process and upon announcement of a proposed policy there should be effective measures to ensure that dissenting views are elicited and given a fair hearing, where this includes utilization of a devil's advocate role, a person or committee charged with challenging the official view. Further, the leaders of the institution should be under a formal obligation to respond publicly, on the merits, to reasonable dissenting voices and should be strictly prohibited from avoiding engagement with the substance of criticisms by impugning the character or credentials of the dissidents.

4. The more important operations of the institution should be reasonably transparent, where this means, inter alia, that the institution should facilitate access to its operations on the part of credible external epistemic communities (such as Non-Governmental Organizations), both for purposes of achieving sociological legitimacy and for effective accountability mechanisms.

5. The institution should be engineered for adaptability in the face of changing challenges over time.

6. There should be periodic, impartial, publicized reviews of institutional performance.

7. There should be a clear delineation of the terms of accountability, including:

(a) specification of the key criteria for evaluating institutional performance, (b) identification of the primary accountability-holders (those who are tasked with applying the criteria for evaluation), and (c) measures to impose costs on relevant institutional agents in the event of a negative evaluation by the primary accountability-holders.

I wish to emphasize that these desiderata are designed not just to facilitate the fair, efficient allocation of vaccines across countries—a topic that has been the main focus of ethical works on the international aspect of the COVID pandemic. They are intended to apply generally to the design of institutions tasked with providing aid to poorer countries, not just in the form of vaccines, but also in therapeutics and in improving medical infrastructures.

FORMAL OR INFORMAL?

The institution should be formal, that is, treaty-based for three reasons: (1) legally binding commitments are, other things being equal, more effective in preventing free-rider and assurance problems and preventing shirking; (2) international treaty law provides procedures for creating institutions that help them achieve sociological legitimacy, which is important for effectiveness, and (3) legal obligations provide clear, public moral coordination points for mobilizing public pressure on governments and pharmaceutical companies.

THE BIG QUESTION: WHY SHOULD RICH COUNTRIES RATIFY SUCH A TREATY?

I remain unconvinced that self-interest on the part of the government leaders of wealthy countries will suffice. They may quite reasonably conclude that they can deal effectively enough with a future pandemic within their countries borders to sustain their own power and avoid criticisms from their citizens while indulging in excessive national partiality. I think it most probable that they will only participate sincerely in the needed institution if prompted to do so by sustained, focused public pressure. I think it is also highly likely that such pressure will not be achieved unless there is a clear moral coordination point: a reasonably detailed outline of what the needed institution would look like along with an understandable explanation of why it is needed. I believe that I have pointed the way toward achieving this first step on the path to institutional innovation.

SIX

Public Health Ideology

The thesis of this chapter is that an ideology common among public health experts has had a negative influence on the development of national COVID-19 policies in the United States and on public health communications regarding those policies. To begin to make the case for this claim, I must first wade into troubled waters by offering a general characterization of ideologies. I do so with some trepidation, because there is much disagreement among theorists of ideologies as to just what an ideology is. The following characterization is broad enough, however, to encompass at least the most common understandings of ideology in the social sciences at present.

Before doing so, a methodological caveat is in order. Ideologies are rarely explicitly formulated; instead, they must be reconstructed. The most important tool of reconstruction is "inference to the best explanation." In other words, if the hypothesis that a group is in the grip of a particular ideology is the best explanation of their dominant discourse and behavior, that is evidence for the existence of the ideology and for the nature of its content. In what follows I attempt to reconstruct a particular public health ideology, or a strain of thinking that may be embedded in a larger, more comprehensive public ideology. I believe that the hypothesis helps to explain both some important elements of the responses of public health authorities to the current pandemic and the reactions of some public health experts to my criticisms of those responses.

An ideology (and here I mean a political ideology) is a systematically interrelated—though not necessarily consistent—set of beliefs, attitudes, and processes for managing beliefs that provide individuals with a common evaluative map of the social world, a map in which groups are typically prominent landmarks, and which includes beliefs about the proper exercise of power, that is, beliefs about when power is legitimate or backed by genuine authority. Ideologies also include belief-management mechanisms, including cognitive-dissonance resolution techniques that allow for the preservation of the ideology's core beliefs in the face of disconfirming evidence, what I call doxastic immune systems. Hence when we say a person is in the grip of an ideology, we imply that her beliefs are excessively rigid, dogmatic, and recalcitrant to correction.

To the extent that ideologies, like maps, simplify various features of the social world, they can be said to misrepresent it. But they may also misrepresent in other ways; for example, by disguising power relations or minimizing power disparities. The map that an ideology presents is not purely descriptive: it includes evaluations of various features of the social world. It is for that reason that ideologies provide practical orientation for individuals in the social world, providing guidance for how they should react to various facts as the ideology presents them. Ideologies serve to coordinate the beliefs and the behavior of those who adhere to them, thereby enabling effective collective action. They also provide a shared identity. Finally, ideologies typically include a moral element: they include moral judgments about who has the authority to wield power and often designate some groups as responsible for what is good about social arrangements and others as responsible for what is wrong with them.

It is important to emphasize that this characterization of ideologies differs significantly from that endorsed by broadly Marxist understandings of ideology. According to some versions of critical theory, it is definitional of ideologies that they function to support oppressive or unjust existing social orders by misrepresenting their nature. To my knowledge this restricted conception of ideology is found nowadays chiefly among some philosophers. It is rejected by most social scientists for a simple reason: they recognize that there are revolutionary ideologies, ideologies that challenge rather than support existing oppressive social orders.

In fact, virtually all social science work on revolutions assigns an explanatory role to ideologies, though there is much disagreement as to the extent of the influence of revolutionary ideologies on the initiation and unfolding of revolutions.[1] An advantage of the characterization of ideology I offered above is that it encompasses both ideologies that challenge the status quo and those that support it.

When I speak of a public health ideology, I mean to call attention to one feature of ideologies: they provide a common identity for a group that is assigned a special role and a special importance in some domain of social life. Thus we can speak of the ideologies of various professional groups. Such ideologies may not be as comprehensive as ideologies that feature a broader identity, but they still serves as simplified evaluative maps of a portion of the social world, namely, that domain in which the professional activity of a particular group takes place. Further, the ideologies of professions not only include beliefs about the rightful exercise of power; they also tend to enhance the power of the particular profession.

My suggestion is that there is something that warrants being called "public health ideology," which includes the following features:

1. The paternalistic/elitist belief that the general population suffers significant cognitive and/or emotional limitations as to their ability to understand and act on the information possessed by the public health experts. Consequently, it is permissible and even obligatory for public health experts to adjust their communications with the public to reflect these limitations. In some cases this will include the deliberate propagation of falsehoods and/or the omission of relevant facts. Such manipulative communication is justified on the grounds that it is for the good of the public—on the assumption that the public health professionals know what that good is.

2. The presumption that proper public health measures involve interventions that affect the entire population. One manifestation of this presumption or rather another component of the ideology that lends support to it is the tendency to invoke the idea of a national health emergency, even in cases in which the emergency is of much narrower scope (for example an emergency for a certain high risk subpopulation).

---

1. See, for example, R. R. Palmer, "The World Revolution of the West: 1763–1801," *Political Science Quarterly* 69, no. 1 (1954): 1–14; Francois Furet, *Interpreting the French Revolution*, translated by the Maison des Sciences de l'Homme (Cambridge: Cambridge University Press, 1981); and Theda Skopcol, *States and Social Revolutions* (Cambridge: Cambridge University Press, 2015) 114, 153–54, 168–71.

3. A tendency to focus only on the direct negative health impact of a pandemic and to endorse policies that only take into account the benefit of preventing that negative impact. This tendency obscures the need for trade-offs and either results in policymakers wholly ignoring the costs of the proposed prevention measures or in their assuming, without good reason, that the benefits of preventing the negative direct health impact of a pandemic obviously outweigh any associated costs. One result of this way of thinking is to assume that the proper goal of policy is not just to mitigate but to eliminate entirely the direct negative health impact of the pandemic— to maximize reduction of one particular risk, rather than to strike an optimal trade-off between mitigating that risk and excessive costs in doing so. Put most simply, this is the tendency to attend only to the supposed benefits of a policy and to disregard the costs.

4. A tendency to make the avoidance of Type 2 errors a priority, which also encourages a failure to take seriously the costs of proposed policies. A Type 2 error occurs when an institution or bureaucracy adopts a policy that produces serious costs or harms. A Type 1 error occurs when an agency adopts a policy that results in loss of some significant benefits. In the case at hand, a Type 2 error occurs when the policymaker fails to prevent avoidable harms to health resulting directly from the pandemic disease. Given the public health expert's conception of her role, what is to be avoided at all costs is the failure to prevent that particular harm. If the role of the public health professional is to prevent harm from diseases, then failure to do so undermines her legitimacy. But prioritizing the avoidance of Type 2 errors distorts policy-making by encouraging disregard for the costs of avoiding that type of error. In effect, the focus on avoiding Type 2 errors obscures the need for trade-offs. Prioritizing the avoidance of Type 2 errors amounts to prioritizing the preservation of the professional's reputation (as the ideology shapes one's conception of it) over the pursuit of the best policy option.

Feature 1 was manifested in U.S. policy. As I noted earlier, Anthony Fauci admitted that he lied to the public, saying that masks weren't necessary, when he knew they were useful tools for reducing transmission of the virus. His justification for this lie was that the public couldn't be trusted to avoid purchasing so many masks that medical workers would not have enough of them. In other words, he assumed that the public wouldn't exercise sufficient self-restraint. Similarly, although public health officials knew that simple cloth masks were ineffective (too porous and not close-fitting enough) they chose to continue to exhort the public to wear masks without specifying that only N95 type masks were effective. Presumably, they thought the public was only capable of understanding the simpler message: wear a mask. Once again, the implied estimate of the abilities of the public is far from flattering. To take another example of paternalistic distrust of the public: consider the fact that the CDC oversold the efficacy of vaccination, frequently stating or implying that it would "prevent" infection or at least "prevent" serious cases of COVID-19. A more accurate statement would have been that vaccination reduces the probability of infection for a short period of time and reduces the probability of serious effects of infection in some individuals. Apparently, CDC spokespersons were afraid that unless they exaggerated the efficacy of vaccination many people would not get vaccinated. Here, too, the assumption was that normal adults are not capable of properly utilizing accurate information.

Like the misrepresentation of public health expertise examined in the preceding chapter, elitist/paternalistic behavior is a wrongful expropriation of power from the public. It deprives people of the opportunity to make responsible decisions by an exercise of power on the part of the professionals that reflects a condescending assumption of their superiority.

I am not assuming that paternalism toward competent adults is never justified (though I think that in the real world, as opposed to philosophers exotic examples, it virtually never is). My point is that an elitist/paternalistic attitude is something like the default view for many public health professionals. This means that they do not trouble themselves to bear the heavy burden of trying to justify paternalism toward normal adults on a case by case basis, but instead too quickly assume the public's incompetence (and their own infallibility).

In Chapter One I observed that feature 2 was on full display in the responses of two public health experts, one American, one British, during the oral discussion after one of my Tanner Lectures at the University of Cambridge in February of 2022. In the lecture, when I suggested that a targeted approach of reducing the risk of death or serious effects of the virus on the high-risk subpopulation might be superior to the shotgun approach of school closings, lockdowns of "non-essential" business, and travel restrictions, both of these public health professionals said I didn't understand what public health is: public health, they said, deals with whole populations.

This reply is patently false. Every year, public health officials single out subpopulations and recommend special interventions for them and only them. For example, people over sixty-five are advised to get shingles vaccinations, and those over sixty-five or who have chronic respiratory ailments are told they should get flu and pneumonia shots. As I suggested in Chapter One, the conception of public health as total population interventions may be a hangover from a time in which most if not all public health measures did affect the whole population (e.g., improvements in food and water sanitation).

Given that the assumption that public health interventions are to be directed at the whole population is not only irrational but also at odds with actual public health practice, how can one explain its persistence? The answer to this question seems to be that public health professionals believe that interventions that apply to everyone foster solidarity, something of great value that is imperiled by the supposedly excessive individualism of developed societies. One wonders, however, whether there are more honest, truth-respecting ways of promoting solidarity,

Element 3 is a bias common to many if not all professions: the tendency to accord excessive importance to the distinctive activity of the profession, the activity that constitutes the professional identity. Thus surgeons tend to see surgery as the solution to all too many problems and military personnel tend to assume that the use of armed force is appropriate in all too many cases. To the extent that health care professionals self-identify as those people who protect the public from diseases, they will tend to focus on the need to prevent diseases and pay too little attention to the costs of prevention. It is revealing that the acronym of the title of agency with the highest authority for responding to pandemics is CDC—standing for Center for Disease Control. The point is that although controlling the spread of a disease is important, it is not all that matters in life. Yet the professional identify of public health agents gives excessive weight to preventing disease, thereby failing to acknowledge the need for trade-offs and assuming in effect that the goal is to achieve maximal protection against the disease rather than optimal protection, given the need to take other goods into account.

Element 4 requires little in the way of elaboration. Giving disproportionate weight to the avoidance of Type 2 errors is ubiquitous in public agencies charged with ensuring safety. Here is a vivid example: in 1982 the FDA announced with considerable satisfaction that it had just approved a cardiac medication that would save 50,000 lives a year.[2] What the announcement did not acknowledge was that this drug had been approved and safely used in Europe for several years. So, another way of characterizing the FDA's behavior was to say that by not approving a safe and efficacious drug they had caused the unnecessary deaths of 50,000 Americans per year for several years. In fact, until recently, the FDA refused to take into account data on drug efficacy and safety produced by similar agencies in Europe, even in cases where their standards were as high or higher than those of the FDA. Apparently more weight was given to avoiding the very low probability of a Type 2 error than to the massive benefits of approving a life-saving drug. As I noted earlier, the incentive for public health professionals is to avoid Type 2 errors, because it is that type of error that is likely to draw the most severe criticism of their performance. Public health ideology puts the stamp of approval on this self-protective behavior by devoting almost exclusive attention to preventing the direct negative health effects of diseases by stopping their spread, thereby contributing to policy decisions that are both irrational and morally irresponsible.

The foregoing discussion of public health ideology is admittedly speculative. This much can be said for it, however: it explains behavior of some public health professionals that, in the absence of an ideological explanation, appears both arbitrary and irrational. The point is that, given the four ideological elements described above, the behavior in question is not unexpected and is *conditionally* rational, that is, rational given the beliefs that constitute the ideology.

2. Wesley G. Pippert, "'New Era' Opens in Treating Heart Disease," *United Press International*. November 25, 1981, https://www.upi.com/Archives/1981/11/25/New-era-opens-in-treating-heart-disease/1126375512400/.

SEVEN

Conclusion

LEADERSHIP AND INSTITUTIONS

It is often said that there was a failure of leadership in responses to the COVID-19 pandemic. That is true, but quite misleading, unless one adds this: failures of leadership were promoted by defective institutions. Even the best institutional innovations do not guarantee success or provide full protection against damage due to poor leadership. At the very least, however, they increase the probability that the most disastrous actions will not be undertaken.

Focusing only on the failings of leaders is not productive. It fosters the illusion that if we had had different leaders all would have been well. It overlooks two crucial facts that are key for providing a better response to the next pandemic: leaders respond to incentives and institutions affect incentives. Too much energy has been expended on vilifying CDC, HHS, and FDA officials and on criticizing presidents Trump and Biden. The key question is this: why did these individuals make the mistakes for which we criticize them?

It is true, of course, that we do need to think hard about how to select better leaders, to improve the mechanisms by which individuals are awarded leadership roles in various domains. But we also need to acknowledge that whether or not the virtues of leadership flourish usually depends in large part on whether institutional incentives support or undermine them.

The task of preparing for the next pandemic is daunting. It is made even more difficult by the fact that the sociological legitimacy of the institutions we must rely on has been seriously undermined due to the institutional failures I have identified. My hope is that if the institutional reforms I have recommended were adopted, this would do something to reduce the legitimacy deficit. They would have this welcome effect if they not only produced better decisions but made the soundness of the decision-making process apparent to the public.

PART II

RESPONSES TO ALLEN BUCHANAN

EIGHT

International Institutions and the Duty to Aid in a Pandemic

The Problem of Noncompliance

CÉCILE FABRE

INTRODUCTION

Allen Buchanan's aim is to offer a blueprint for institutional reforms which, on his view, would help us prepare better for the next pandemic. Unless we take a long hard look at domestic and international responses to the COVID-19 pandemic, he argues, we are condemned to repeating the mistakes we made then.

Buchanan's essays, which grow out of his Tanner Lectures, are an indictment of steps taken to fight the COVID-19 pandemic by U.S. institutions such as the CDC, the FDA, and the Trump and Biden administrations, wealthy countries in the Global North, and international institutions such as the World Health Organization (WHO). In his account, the main domestic responses to the pandemic (mass vaccination and nationwide lockdowns) were marred by serious institutional failures. Those failures are traceable to undue confidence in the supposedly expert judgment of health officials, undue interference by political officials in the design of health policy, and unwillingness on the part of both health and political officials to consider alternative viewpoints. Moreover, countries in the Global North unnecessarily hoarded millions of vaccine doses at the expense of countries in the Global South, and international institutions' attempts to distribute vaccines fairly were ineffective.

I do not dispute (who would?) that a number of mistakes were made, both nationally and internationally, but I simply do not share Buchanan's wholesale condemnation of mass vaccination and lockdowns. This is well-trodden territory, which I will not revisit. Instead, I focus on his proposal for international institutional reforms and on the moral framework which underpins it.

THE DEMANDS OF JUSTICE

In Buchanan's account, individuals owe at least two pre-institutional moral duties to others, which are relevant here. For ease of reference, I shall call those duties "Buchanan-duties." First, individuals are under a duty to prevent and mitigate serious harms to others, including to distant strangers, subject to a no-undue-costs proviso. The duty to rescue is a duty of justice; as such, it is owed to specific individuals, and it is enforceable. Unlike, say, the duty not to kill, it is often highly indeterminate with respect to its content. True, if I am faced with the proverbial scenario of a child drowning in a shallow pond and if I can wade in and rescue it at little cost to myself, it is crystal clear that I am under a duty to do so. More often than not, however, one cannot infer from the claim that we are under a duty to rescue others from unwarranted harm, that we are under a duty to fund certain kinds of healthcare treatment rather than others, to prioritise the needs of the very young over the needs of the very old, to nationalise critical infrastructure or to leave it to private actors subject to various kinds of constraints—and so on. Moreover, when discharging the duty requires a collaborative effort, merely to say that there is such a duty does not tell us what is a fair allocation of the costs of fulfilling it. As a result, it is all too easy for individuals to fail to comply, or to misfire when they attempt to help. If I do not know what I should do to help you, I am likely not to do anything, or to direct my efforts to those who in fact need it the least. Hence the second Buchanan duty of justice: it is a duty to set up institutions that will "(1) identify specific duty bearers and right-holders (2) in such a way as to distribute the costs of rescuing large numbers of people in a fair manner, and (3) can include mechanisms for compliance with the duties they specify, either through the threat of penalties for noncompliance or rewards for compliance."[1]

I am in broad agreement with Buchanan's account of what justice requires of us. I also agree with him that our duties of justice do not stop at national borders: we owe them not merely to our compatriots, but to distant strangers as well. The only justifications for prioritising our compatriots lie, first, in a general fiduciary obligation to prioritise them under conditions of both *dire* emergency and severe uncertainty as to how bad the situation is; second, past that stage, in the instrumental benefit of dividing the labor of preventing and mitigating harms between states. Crucially, however, the division of labor argument does not justify unconstrained partiality for one's compatriots.[2]

To be clear, as Paul Tucker shows in his contribution to this volume, we need not appeal to those two pre-institutional moral duties of justice in order to get to Buchanan's key conclusions. A properly reconstructed political morality, along the lines of David Hume's and Bernard Williams's, supports the view that public officials ought (not least for prudential, incentive-based reasons) to deploy adequate justifications for their chosen policies (particularly coercively enforced policy). It also supports the view that states ought to cooperate with one another to mitigate pandemic related harms globally. Nevertheless, and not just for the sake of argument, I accept Buchanan's starting point.

In my response, I examine cases in which states, citizenries, and other relevantly implicated actors—such as pharmaceutical companies and civil society actors—are derelict in those duties of justice. Compliance failures raise at least two questions. The first and familiar question is the question of enforcement. While Buchanan believes that duties of justice are enforceable, he does not explore in depth what enforcement measures are morally justified. The second, less familiar question, asks whether compliant actors are under a moral obligation to take up the slack created by noncompliant actors—in other words, to do more than their fair share. My aim is not to show (as philosophers are wont to do) where Buchanan's

1. See Chapter Five, page 67, this volume.

2. For recent defences of the global scope of the duty to rescue others from pandemic-related harms, against the view that states are permitted to hoard vaccines in excess of what their population needs, see esp. Ezekiel J. Emanuel, Allen Buchanan, Cécile Fabre et al., "On the Ethics of Vaccine Nationalism: The Case for the Fair Priority for Residents Framework," *Ethics & International Affairs* 35, no. 4 (2021): 543–62; Ezekiel J. Emanuel, Allen Buchanan, Cécile Fabre et al., "An Ethical Framework for Global Vaccine Allocation," *Science* 369, no. 6509 (2020): 1309–12.

account has gone wrong. Rather, it is to build on it, by sketching out lines of inquiry that are worth pursuing.

ENFORCING DUTIES

Suppose that some actor is derelict in its Buchanan-duties. For example, the government of a very wealthy country—call it Blue—takes an extreme nationalist view and refuses to transfer resources to any of the poorest countries in the world towards mitigating COVID-related harms, even though a modest amount of redistribution would not jeopardise its ability to cater for the needs of its own population. Or, more interestingly, Blue agrees that it ought to be only moderately partial towards its own citizens, but claims it has a very clear understanding of what its global duties are and refuses to cooperate with other governments, charities, pharmaceutical companies, etc. As a result, Blue ends up doing worse at the bar of justice than if it had cooperated with those actors. What, if anything, may other actors—such as other states, international institutions, or indeed private actors—do to enforce Blue's duty to rescue?

In the philosophical literature on enforcement and compliance in the context of global politics, the focus is on whether and how to enforce duties not to harm—negative duties, as they are sometimes called. For example, suppose that Blue mounts a military invasion of Red's territory, in violation of the norm against unwarranted aggression on another country's territorial integrity and political sovereignty. The question then arises as to what third parties (notably the international community) are morally allowed to do in response: come to Red's defence by supplying troops and/or equipment, impose economic sanctions on Blue, expel the latter's diplomats, etc.[3]

However, Buchanan-duties (as defended in this volume) are duties to *do* something—or positive duties. Yet there is very little discussion, in global ethics, of what we may permissibly do to enforce compliance with those duties, in fact, whether we may even permissibly do anything at all other than issue condemnatory statements. Thus, while it is standard to

3. See, e.g., Joy Gordon, "A Peaceful, Silent, Deadly Remedy: The Ethics of Economic Sanctions," *Ethics & International Affairs* 13 (March 1999): 123–42; Robert W. McGee, "The Ethics of Economic Sanctions," *Economic Affairs* 23, no. 4 (2003): 41–45; Robert A. Pape, "Why Economic Sanctions Do Not Work," *International Security* 22, no. 2 (1997): 90–136; James Pattison, *The Alternatives to War—from Sanctions to Nonviolence* (Oxford: Oxford University Press, 2018); Cécile Fabre, *Economic Statecraft:Human Rights, Sanctions and Conditionality* (Cambridge, MA: Harvard University Press, 2018); "Military Intervention in Inter-State Conflicts," *Social Philosophy & Policy* (forthcoming 2024).

say that military attacks on Red's territorial integrity provide a just cause for defensive military action or economic sanctions, it is *absolutely not* standard to say, or even to reflect, on whether wrongful failures, at the bar of justice, to prevent and mitigate grievous harms such as the harms of global poverty or of a pandemic warrant these sorts of measures.[4]

When we reflect on enforcing Blue's negative duties not to harm, we might want, and are *pro tanto* morally allowed, to *incapacitate* Blue by, for example, attacking its troops. We might want, and are *pro tanto* morally allowed, to *deter* Blue from going any further by, for example, imposing economic sanctions on its regime. We might want, and are *pro tanto* morally allowed, to *induce* Blue to withdraw its troops by, for example, offering something in return such as territorial concessions, the promise of a trade deal, or purchasing natural resources from it rather than from other parties.

Let us see, then, whether the tripartite distinction between incapacitation, deterrence, and inducements is of any use with respect to the enforcement of Buchanan-duties. Consider first enforcement by incapacitation. That is not promising: if your aim is to get someone to do something, such as providing resources and cooperating with other duty-bearers, incapacitating them is not the right way to go about it.

Enforcement by deterrence is more promising. Consider the welfare state. It renders determinate via laws and law-like directives, and in particular taxation law, our duty to prevent and mitigate harm to fellow citizens. If I willfully fail to pay the taxes which I am under a legal duty to pay, I am subject to criminal sanctions. On the deterrence view, criminal sanctions are morally justified as a means both to deter me from breaking the law again, and to deter other putative lawbreakers.

By analogy, then, we must set up institutions with enforcement mechanisms meant to deter actors (states, charities, pharmaceutical companies, etc.) from breaking the rules which those institutions will have also established to deal with the next pandemic. That said, note, first, that this will not work against Blue's refusal to cooperate in the establishment *de novo* of those institutions—in other words, prior to rules being in existence. That is a serious limitation of deterrence in this context.

Note, second, that deterrent measures will need to be fit for the task of getting Blue to comply with its duty to prevent and mitigate pandemic-related harms as well as its duty to cooperate towards the ongoing

---

4. For the view that culpable failures to alleviate severe poverty may constitute a just cause for war, see Cécile Fabre, *Cosmopolitan War* (Oxford: Oxford University Press, 2012), chap. 3; Victor Tadros, "Resource Wars," *Law and Philosophy* 33 (2014): 361–89.

functioning of those institutions. Some of those measures are likely to be very different from deterrent measures aimed at forestalling military aggression. What might be effective, necessary, and proportionate as a deterrent against aggression, might fail on all three counts as a deterrent against breaking the pandemic-related rules. This is not to imply that deterrence is not a useful normative framework for tackling noncompliance with Buchanan-duties; it is merely to suggest that the issue warrants further investigation.

Consider finally enforcement by inducement. There is scant literature on the ethics of offering inducements as a means to get agents to fulfil their duties, even though, in practice, this is what aid conditionality sometimes amounts to.[5] We might want to distinguish two cases. In the first case, Blue has an independent claim to what we would offer as an inducement. For example, Blue does have a legitimate title to a parcel of territory over which some other state exercises *de facto* control. The important question here is whether Blue has forfeited its title by failing to fulfill its Buchanan-duties. If it has, then it is morally appropriate to make the offer of that territory conditional upon its fulfilling its duties. But if it has not forfeited its title merely by dint of refusing to fulfil its Buchanan-duties, then we ought not to make the retrocession of that territory conditional on Blue's compliance.

In the second case, Blue has no moral claim to what would induce it to fulfill its Buchanan-duties. Suppose, for example, that Blue would (in the next pandemic) distribute surplus vaccine doses to poor countries instead of hoarding them, so long as other countries buy natural gas from it—at greater cost to them than if they bought on other markets. Blue is not entitled to demand that other states call on its reserves of gas to meet their energy needs in general, and at those costs in particular. The question here is what those third parties must do in response to Blue's illicit demands, in fulfilment of their duty to prevent and mitigate harms to distant strangers. On the one hand, we could argue that they are under a duty to shoulder the costs of enforcing Blue's own duty by offering Blue that to which it is not entitled anyway. However, this seems doubly unfair: not only do third parties have to divest themselves of resources which they might need (namely, the resources needed to pay the difference between buying Blue's gas and buying cheaper gas elsewhere), and unnecessarily

---

5. The literature on the ethics of aid conditionality is seriously underdeveloped. For an exception, see Fabre, *Economic Statecraft*, chaps. 4–5.

so; in addition, Blue gets more than it is owed, as a "reward" for not doing its duty. On the other hand, we could argue that third parties are under a moral duty to take up the slack, by doing Blue's share.

TAKING UP THE SLACK

Suppose, then, that Blue fails to do its fair share of what is required to set up and maintain the institutions we need to deal with the next pandemic. Or suppose that those institutions have determined that Blue's general duty to prevent and mitigate pandemic-related harms consists in doing w, while Green, Red, Yellow, etc., are each under duties to do x, y, and z. Blue refuses to do w. Are Green, Red, Yellow, etc., under a duty to step into the breach—in other words, to do more than x, y, z?

Some philosophers argue that they are not: they are under a duty to do their fair share, and no more—when what constitutes their fair share is based on the assumption that all duty-bearers comply. On this view, if it has been determined that wealthy states must together subsidise the cost of vaccines worldwide, and if Blue refuses to comply, other duty-bearers are not under a duty to do more than they already do. Specifically, pharmaceutical companies are not under duties to sell at a loss; and other wealthy states are not under a duty to pay Blue's share of total subsidies. This is because it would be unfair to insist that they take up the slack.[6]

The unfairness objection to the duty to take up the slack is misguided, as I believe Buchanan would agree. At any rate, his account does support such a duty. Suppose that Green could do more than x, thus taking up the slack, *and* that it would not be unreasonably costly for it to do so. Unfair? Perhaps. But it doesn't follow that Green is not under such a duty. Returning to the duty to enforce compliance, it *is* costly, and those costs are unfair. Think, in the domestic context, of having to fund the police and to maintain a justice system. Think, in the foreign policy case, of having to maintain armies and to supply weapons. The rationale for those institutions is precisely that they serve to enforce moral duties such as duties not to kill, not to rape, not to steal, not to invade another country, and so on. I take it for granted that we are under a duty to shoulder those costs,

---

6. See in particular Liam B. Murphy, "The Demands of Beneficence," *Philosophy & Public Affairs* 22, no. 4 (1993): 267–92. For very good critical discussions, see Anja Karnein, "Putting Fairness in Its Place: Why There Is a Duty to Take up the Slack," *The Journal of Philosophy* 111, no. 11 (2014): 593–607; Zofia Stemplowska, "Doing More Than One's Fair Share," *Critical Review of International Social and Political Philosophy* 19, no. 5 (2016): 591–608. Karnein and Stemplowska both think that there is a duty to take up the slack. I am largely in agreement with them.

in response to wrongdoers' dereliction, *notwithstanding the fact that it is unfair of wrongdoers to put us in that position*. If this is correct, one cannot appeal to the unfairness of having to pay for wrongdoers' dereliction of duty as grounds for rejecting a duty to take up the slack. Moreover, taking up the slack is less unfair than enforcing Blue's compliance via induce-ments: instead of diverting much needed additional resources towards Blue, which does not have a claim to them, we divert them towards those who need them. To put the point slightly differently: what matters, for determining what Green and others ought to do in response to Blue's der-eliction, is their moral relationship *to victims of pandemic-related harms*, not to other duty-bearers. What they owe to victims, all things considered, is limited by what costs they may be reasonably be expected to bear. The mere fact of others' noncompliance is irrelevant.

To be sure, there might be good reasons not to institutionalise the duty to take up the slack. If institutions specifically determine that, in the event of Blue not doing w, Green, Red, and Yellow will be asked respectively to contribute x^+, y^+, and z^+, Blue will have a strong incentive not to do its share. Here too Buchanan would agree. As he rightly notes, and as Tucker convincingly shows at greater length, institution-design must be sensitive to incentives. If institutionalising a duty (of any kind) gives rise to moral hazard, and if we cannot also institutionalise effective deterrent measures against slackers, then we have *pro tanto* reasons not to institutionalise. Whether institutionalisation would have those justice-impairing conse-quences is a matter for empirical investigation. Crucially, however, this concession to incentives does not undermine the claim that there is a *pro tanto* moral duty to take up the slack in the first instance.

CONCLUSION

I have sketched out some thoughts one might have, in the light of Buchan-an's account of what we ought to do to prepare for the next pandemic, about the problem of noncompliance. The main lesson to draw from my remarks is twofold. First, there is need for more work, in global ethics, on the difficult issue of enforcing compliance with positive duties to pro-vide assistance. Second, thinking about enforcement sheds some light on the issue of whether or not there is a duty to take up the slack created by noncompliers.

Although my remarks are set in the specific context of the pandemic, they have purchase in other contexts as well. So does Buchanan's account of justice. The two duties that it defends apply not only to pandemic-related harms but also to any kind of harm the prevention and mitigation of which calls for a global response—such as climate change and military conflicts. Whatever one thinks of his empirical claims about some of the steps taken by many national and international institutions during the COVID-19 pandemic, he has made a significant contribution to debates on the need for reforms.

NINE

The Challenge of Incentives-Values Compatibility in International Cooperation

PAUL TUCKER

Allen Buchanan's Tanner Lectures address how political-ethical issues bear on policy choices and the design of institutions for avoiding and containing pandemics, understood as epidemics that rapidly spread across borders, showing no respect for the territorial organisation of political communities. Some will be roused to reasoned fury by the position he takes on the policies adopted during COVID-19 by many Western nations, and on the performance of various U.S. agencies. Others may applaud. I do not engage with that, partly because many of Buchanan's views on recent events are, to my mind, orthogonal to the important questions he raises about how to think about crisis management practices and institutions. Better justifications were needed for domestic emergency policies, he says, and institutional reform is needed both at home and internationally. Both are hard to quarrel with.

More important, I agree with Buchanan that it is useful to frame the issues in terms of legitimacy and legitimation. But if my observations have a common theme, it is that the pre-political morality deployed by Buchanan—the language of general moral duties of justice—is not necessary to reach conclusions similar to his. That matters because, if so, it means it might be useful to frame some of the arguments in terms more likely to make sense to the concerns and circumstances of those—policymakers and citizens—who need to be persuaded for any meaningful reforms to stand a chance. The point is not that morality does not matter but that there is value in exploring, in the spirit of Bernard Williams's late-in-life political philosophy, whether it can be found within the practices and circumstances of politics itself, viewed as collective actions aimed at achieving and sustaining basic order and conditions for cooperation without excessive coercion and conflict.[1] Seen thus, Buchanan's prescriptions for a new international health regime face another hurdle: geopolitics.[2]

JUSTIFICATION OF CRISIS MANAGEMENT AS CENTRAL TO LEGITIMACY

Buchanan argues that the authorities should have done more to justify their pandemic responses given they entailed restricting people's liberties. They were under a moral obligation to provide such a justification given the respect each person is due by virtue of their being moral equals.[3]

Buchanan is surely right in pinpointing the vital importance of justification. Where the response to a disaster is dramatic, power holders need to explain themselves for a whole gamut of reasons. Crises almost by definition violate a political community's sense of how things should be and of how things should be done (the good and the right). They damage perceptions of the competence and, sometimes, the decency of government. Where a disaster exposes serious inadequacies in government, authorities need to explain why the failings are not pathological to the system of government, and how they can be remedied in ways that do not add to the problem by violating norms for how things should be done. Crises and crisis measures accordingly put pressure on any demand for legitimation.

We can, however, explain that general demand without levering off a pre-political moral principle. As Williams argued, any attempt to achieve and sustain order poses a Basic Legitimation Demand (BLD): that those exercising a formal monopoly over means of coercion—or, it should

---

1. Bernard Williams, *In the Beginning Was the Deed: Realism and Moralism in Political Argument,* selected, edited, and with an introduction by Geoffrey Hawthorne (Princeton: Princeton University Press, 2005).

2. As such, this short commentary extends the applications of the framework in my *Global Discord: Values and Power in a Fractured World Order* (Princeton: Princeton University Press, 2022).

3. See Chapter One, page 15, and pages 21–23, this volume.

be added, any type of formalised hierarchical authority—need to offer an account of why it should be accepted (given reasonably available alternatives). As he puts it, otherwise the solution becomes part of the problem.[4]

What Williams did not go on to address is why, other than for the kind of pre-political moral reasons he was trying to avoid, rulers would in practice choose to offer any such justification. The obvious answer is that otherwise resistance, or the prospect of resistance, active or passive, threatens to reduce their (risk-adjusted) returns from ruling. Legitimation norms arise and persist where Williams's demand for legitimation reaches an equilibrium with the Basic Legitimation Supply I am positing.[5]

Any such functional account of legitimation does not preclude, and indeed is fortified by, actors coming to internalise legitimation as having intrinsic value. But the moral value accorded to legitimation (and its normative outputs) does not need to be rooted in some unique deeper value (say, a pre-political moral right to equal political respect). It can be enough to excavate its (and their) functional purpose, to find that that purpose withstands critical scrutiny, and to reflect that the practice serves a number of moral purposes for the political community, including helping to hold it together during trials and tribulations. On that account, as much as with Buchanan's, crisis managers, great or small, ex ante and ex post, are always partly stewards of political order.

Whatever the routes to that banal conclusion, it opens a door to elaborating on Buchanan's thoughts on what within-crisis explanations and justifications look like in ways that might test some of his verdicts on the handling of COVID-19.

EXPLAINING AND JUSTIFYING CRISIS MEASURES

Good policy is almost always conditional. Broadly, it has the following structure: given the policymaker's current epistemic understanding of the problem (E) and its objective (O), the chosen response is XYZ.

The epistemic diagnosis itself has three components. The first is an understanding of the nature of the shock (whether, say, a virus or bacteria is causing sickness); call that Es. Second is the understanding of how the shock will be propagated through the relevant domain (does the virus spread via the air or touch, how deadly is it, etc.), designated Ep. And the

---

4. Williams, "Realism and Moralism in Political Theory," in *In The Beginning Was the Deed*, 5.

5. Argued more fully in Paul Tucker, "Basic Legitimation Supply and Bernard Williams' Political Theory" (forthcoming).

third epistemic element is the policymakers' (and others') understanding of the efficacy of their instruments for containing or offsetting the propagation of the shock, and how those effects are transmitted through the system, Ei. A policymaker could have a firm epistemic grip on one of those but not the others.

To make sense to the public, the structure of crisis-management communications needs to track that decision-making structure: viz, "our understanding of this problem is E and our goal is O, so we are responding with XYZ." There might need to be changes in the policy response (XYZ) as the crisis manager's diagnosis (E) develops. Crudely, there is a need for something akin to Bayesian updating.

This simple schema helps bring out what is going on when, during a drawn-out crisis, such as the recent pandemic, the policy response alters. The most problematic kind of course change is made when O and E (in all three dimensions) are (truly) unchanged. Is interest-group politics the reason? Properly conditional statements of policy at the outset might help expose that, and so deter it.[6]

A second type of evolving public communication holds Es and Ep constant but changes O and therefore XYZ; i.e., the wrong conclusions, at every level, had previously been reached from the diagnosis of the shock and its propagation. That is clearly a U-turn of a special kind. Putting flawed reasoning to one side, it is most likely explained by policymakers changing their view on what their policy instruments can realistically achieve (Ei); perhaps they were turning out to be weaker (or stronger) than thought, or came on stream faster or slower than expected, and so the goalposts had to be moved.

A third type of communications shift—frequent in real crises—is that E has changed, and so XYZ must change to pursue a maintained objective. This is not a U-turn, but will often look like it unless the conditionality of the initial and ongoing response was reasonably clear to begin with. This third hazard is especially important when policymakers' initial understanding is limited but includes a notion of what the maximum plausible damage might be, together with certainty that they do not have a ready solution to hand; for example, it is a deadly virus, they do not know how deadly, but they know for sure a vaccine or cure will take many months or years. In those circumstances, if the maximum plausible damage is grossly

6. Complete openness might, however, be perverse if it would compromise national security or prompt panic.

severe, one possible response is to take dramatic action that attempts to freeze the propagation of the problem. That can help make sense of an early lockdown in a pandemic, just as it explains F. D. Roosevelt's bank holiday—effectively shutting down the U.S. economy, other than via barter—during the 1930s banking crisis. Time is bought to think about what to do. When the policymaker introduces new measures, they need to explain them in terms of their better understanding of the underlying problem(s) and/or the effectiveness of their instruments. By revealing the structure of the argument, this sheds light on how to debate Buchanan's criticisms of policy on lockdowns and vaccines.

Those parables point to another precept. Throughout a crisis, policymakers need to convey the degree of uncertainty they have about their understanding of what is going on, glossed with explanations of whether they view the risks around their (for the time being) central view as symmetric or asymmetric. *Pace* Buchanan,[7] sensible policymakers and technical advisors (called "experts" in the main lecture) avoid claiming to know more than they do. Professed ignorance with credible explanations of likely severity might sometimes help warrant dramatic actions policymakers take (at least initially).

INTERNATIONAL COOPERATION AND REFORM

Away from domestic policy, Buchanan holds that that well-resourced states have moral Duties of Justice to help poorer and weaker states cope with pandemics; and that the vehicle should be a regime, framed by an international treaty and administered by an international organisation, that turns those moral duties into concrete positive-law obligations and rights. In making his case, Buchanan starts by arguing against both an inward-looking (illiberal) nationalism, and also a philosophical cosmopolitanism centred on individuals as individuals, abstracted from any kind of local community. There are sometimes moral duties to help outsiders but they can sometimes be trumped by duties at home. Again, I want to argue, we can get there without summoning a pre-political morality.

Establishing and maintaining basic order, even locally, is a challenge. Doing so in ways that people can go along with, and so involving legitimate authority of some kind, is an achievement—a political achievement. It is best not to take that for granted, and to have some kind of handle on what it involves in particular concrete circumstances. The legitimation

---

7. See Chapter One, pages 12–14, this volume.

justifications that we receive, reflect on, and in turn offer to each other are, in most cases, partly a product of history: they are path dependent as social scientists would say, or for "now and around here" in the words of Bernard Williams.[8] If something like that is a fact of the world, and if achieving order, safety, protection, and some degree of intracommunal trust provides conditions for cooperation on more ambitious collective endeavours—meeting shared problems and threats, securing opportunities—we need to recognise that that is no small matter, which is why Williams dubbed it the First Political Question. Among other things, it implies that a political community should be careful not to jeopardise local order and legitimacy when contemplating whether or how to help (or intervene in the life of) a separate community. Concretely, taking Britain as an example, during the COVID-19 pandemic it would have been reckless for any UK government to provide help overseas if that plausibly would have led to the National Health Service (NHS) falling apart. That is because, since World War II, the NHS has been an important part of whatever holds Britain together.

Instrumental Reasons to Cooperate with Other States on Pandemics

It matters whether that middling approach[9]—entailing a presumptive respect for other states, and degrees of amity varying with how far their own legitimation norms include something like our notion of the most basic rights—can find reasons to cooperate on preventing and containing pandemics without resorting to pre-political moral duties. Without at all wanting to argue that only instrumental reasons matter, it is obvious that rich states do have instrumental reasons to cooperate (if they can). Three will suffice, in no particular order.

First, if a virus is left unconstrained abroad, we are more likely to import mutations even when we have neutralised its primary form. Bluntly, short of attempted autarky, we are hardly safe from plague if it rampages elsewhere.

Second, uncontrolled disease in poor states might prompt massive numbers of people to flee, leaving richer countries struggling to cope. This seems like an unpleasant thought, even one motivated by the option of leaving others to die in order to preserve our way of life, but that is not its substance or spirit. Helping the people of other states to survive means

8. Williams, "Realism and Moralism," 8.

9. It might be cast as moderate cosmopolitanism or as a liberal nationalism, or somewhere in-between.

helping them to survive as political communities, recognising the value to both them and us of their own achievement of local order with their own ways of life.

That relates to the third reason to help. With today's superpowers embarked upon what is likely to be a decades-long contest, we, the rich liberal democracies of the world, need all the friends we can find, and certainly cannot afford to alienate poorer peoples by leaving them to collapse from curable disease. The geopolitical predicament of the superpowers gives them each incentives to compete to help less well-off societies.[10]

There is nothing here, note, about helping others in order to preserve foreign markets for our businesses. Even so, there is not much morally admirable about those three arguments, other than their sensitivity to the precious achievement by other states of legitimate local political order. But moral virtue is not the point here. The point is that we do not need to posit a general duty of justice to (try to) do good in the world in the face of pandemic risks. We have reason enough to do so. The greater question, on this line of argument, is not whether we should seek to cooperate but, rather, whether there is much hope of being able to cooperate.

Institutions as Commitment Devices: Incentive Compatibility

Having reasons to act in a certain way and sticking to them are often different things. Actors' preferences might not be stable, or there might be reasons to depart from plans even with unchanged objectives (a time-inconsistency problem, in the jargon of social scientists). Formalised institutions seek to mitigate such commitment problems by making promises overt, public, detailed, and (sometimes) consequential.

Analytically, there is nothing new about this. Whereas for modern Hobbesians promises merely relocate a collective-action problem, Hume showed long ago that they can help to change the stakes. Even if A and B are choosing whether to cooperate on something that has no material externalities, so that others don't care about the outcome as such, the rest of us might care greatly if we discover that A does not abide by a formal promise (a pact) because, in quite different situations, we might care whether A keeps promises.[11]

10. Of course, if the competition gets out of control, with each side spending far more than needed to make or keep friends, the possibility of cooperation reenters as they have reason to coordinate on spending less. A broad analogy would be the Soviets and the U.S. eventually trying to curb their arms race during the old Cold War.

11. David Hume, *A Treatise of Human Nature*, ed. L. A. Selby-Bigge and P. H. Nidditch, 2nd edition (Oxford: Oxford University Press, 1978 [1739]), Book III.

Raising the stakes in that broad way is the purpose of many international organisations. Whether they work—in the sense of establishing practices that persist in equilibrium—depends on whether they are incentive-compatible for all the key actors.[12] Incentive-compatible things happen. Incentive-incompatible things do not. That makes the design of any institution demanding. Stigma and repeat interactions help, but might not always suffice.

This is illustrated by the vital question raised by Cécile Fabre's parallel commentary on Buchanan's lecture: if and when a state fails to make its agreed contribution to a cooperative pandemic (or other such) scheme, should the others somehow enforce compliance, or instead contribute more themselves? Fabre's acute question exposes how difficult it is to keep (some variant of) realism at bay when thinking about international regimes, which another of Hume's penetrating insights will underline.

International Cooperation When Hume's Knaves are Competing Giants

Hume's "sensible knave" free rides on the collective efforts of others when confident that they will not follow suit.[13] After arguing that reason alone will not move the knave (anticipating basic rationalist game theory), Hume says the only remedy is social condemnation—a kind of ostracism that seeks to generate shame, or at least deter others. As already argued, the force of the sanction likely depends on most people in the community having internalised the values that some practice or institution supposedly exists to serve (or instantiate).

But things are more complicated in an international setting. Political communities interact with each other in unfriendly as well as friendly ways, and so the problem of order rears its head among communities as well as within them. Any solution to what is, in effect, the First *International* Political Question brings its own legitimation problem.[14] That being so, there is obviously scope for tension between vertical local legitimation norms and the horizontal international legitimation norms that have emerged from and help underpin an international order. When an

12. I pressed that at Buchanan's Tanner Lecture, and I am glad he makes more of it here. For a formally rigorous account of institutions, see Roger B. Myerson, "Fundamental Theory of Institutions: A Lecture in Honor of Leo Hurwicz," The Hurwicz Lecture, presented at the North American Meetings of the Econometric Society, University of Minnesota, June 22, 2006. See https://home.uchicago.edu/~rmyerson/research/hurwicz.pdf.

13. David Hume, *An Enquiry Concerning the Principles of Morals*, ed. J. B. Schneewind (Indianapolis: Hackett, 1983 [1751]), IX.22, 81.

14. Tucker, *Global Discord*, 299–307.

order has been long-lived, whether via a balance of power or hegemonic leadership, some kind of equilibrium reconciling norms, interests, and power will have been reached. But the rise of a new power perturbs the equilibrium.

Hume's parable accordingly becomes less useful because it implicitly assumes all the actors are roughly the same size (in terms of social position, influence, or power); in international relations, that is not so. There are a few giants, and the calculus works differently if they act, in effect, as giant knaves. In today's world, we see that Russia, a major nuclear power, simply does not care about moral or social sanction from the "international community."

But the People's Republic of China and the United States provide more important cases, as illustrated by a story about the World Health Organization (WHO). In 2002–2003 the Beijing government omitted to inform the WHO about the SARS outbreak in its territory. Trying to learn lessons, in 2007 the WHO strengthened its rules, requiring reporting within twenty-four hours of any events that constitute a health emergency of international concern. But in late 2019 and early 2020, Beijing failed to alert the WHO to the outbreak of COVID. The new rule made no difference.

There is a parallel here with the interesting idea that any pact to address climate change could be enforced via the trade regime. Roughly, if a state failed to comply with its climate obligations, other states would be free to impose trade barriers (which are usually barred other than for reasons of national security). In the jargon of game theory, this would embed the climate regime within the trade regime. The problem is that, today, the trade game is embedded in the security game. That is to say that those deciding whether or not to impose tariffs would have to weigh, seriously and carefully, whether doing so might exacerbate the tense security environment, even provoking aggressive action of some kind. It matters, further, that unlike Moscow and Washington during the old Cold War, today's two all-purpose superpowers have not agreed upon de-escalation protocols.

SUMMING UP

Buchanan makes a strong case for international cooperation to combat pandemics. I have argued that the case for such cooperation does not have to mobilise a deontic general Duty of Justice. We have strong local reasons to offer help. How easy it will be to do so in cooperation during geopolitical stress is open to doubt. The international social norms that, in the background, do a lot of work in oiling the wheels of international organisations are themselves now contested among the very powers vital for peaceful coexistence. That does not vanquish the case for helping, but it complicates it.

It is important and intriguing, finally, to note that pre-political moral reasons to help poorer and weaker states might matter more when trials and tribulations visited upon other, especially distant peoples are extremely unlikely to spill over to us in any way. That might need something closer to a purely moral argument, but it would still need to be one that made sense to the citizens of rich democracies in their particular political circumstances.

CONTRIBUTORS

Allen Buchanan is Laureate Professor of Philosophy and Freedom Center Research Professor at the University of Arizona and James B. Duke Distinguished Professor Emeritus, Duke University. He has published extensively in bioethics, political philosophy, and the philosophy of international law. Buchanan has served as a staff member or consultant on all of the U.S. Presidential Bioethics Commissions, as a member of the Advisory Council for the National Human Genome Research Project, and as a member of the Secretary of Health and Human Services Committee on Genetic Testing. His most recent book is *Our Moral Fate: Evolution and the Escape from Tribalism.* Allen Buchanan's Tanner Lecture was presented in 2022 at the University of Cambridge.

Cécile Fabre is professor of political philosophy and Senior Research Fellow in Politics, All Souls College, Oxford. She is the author, most recently, of *Spying Through a Glass Darkly: The Ethics of Espionage and Counter-Intelligence.*

Paul Tucker is Research Fellow at the Mossavar-Rahmani Center in the John F. Kennedy School of Government at Harvard University. His most recent book is *Global Discord: Values and Power in a Fractured World Order.* .

TRUSTEES OF THE TANNER
LECTURES ON HUMAN VALUES

CHANCELLOR CAROL CHRIST
University of California, Berkeley

VICE CHANCELLOR DEBORAH PRENTICE AND JEREMY ADELMAN
University of Cambridge

PRESIDENT C. ALAN SHORT AND SLAINE CAMPBELL
Clare Hall, Cambridge

PRESIDENT CLAUDINE GAY AND CHRISTOPHER AFENDULIS
Harvard University

PRINCIPAL NICK LEIMU-BROWN AND ROOSA LEIMU-BROWN
Linacre College, Oxford

PRESIDENT SANTA ONO AND GWENDOLYN YIP
University of Michigan

VICE CHANCELLOR IRENE TRACEY AND MYLES ALLEN
University of Oxford

PRESIDENT CHRISTOPHER EISGRUBER AND LORI MARTIN
Princeton University

PRESIDENT MARC TESSIER-LAVIGNE AND MARY HYNES
Stanford University

PRESIDENT TAYLOR RANDALL AND JANET RANDALL
University of Utah

PRESIDENT PETER SALOVEY AND MARTA MORET
Yale University

STEPHEN TANNER IRISH
Chair, O. C. Tanner Board of Directors

DAVID AND TERI PETERSEN
CEO, O. C. Tanner Company

MARK MATHESON AND JENNIFER FALK
Director, Tanner Lectures

INDEX